Career Planning for Everyone in the NHS

THE TOOLKIT

Edited by

Ruth Chambers

General Practitioner
Clinical Dean
Staffordshire University
Head of Stoke-on-Trent Teaching PCT Programme

With contributions from

Wendy Garcarz
Neil Houston
Anne Longbottom
Kay Mohanna
Fiona Taylor

Radcliffe Publishing
Oxford • Seattle

Radcliffe Publishing Ltd
18 Marcham Road
Abingdon
Oxon OX14 1AA
United Kingdom

www.radcliffe-oxford.com
Electronic catalogue and worldwide online ordering facility.

British Library Cataloguing in Publication Data

A catalogue record for this book is available from the British Library.

ISBN 185775 663 0

Typeset by Advance Typesetting Ltd, Oxford
Printed and bound by TJ International Ltd, Padstow, Cornwall

Contents

About the authors

Ruth Chambers has been a GP for more than 20 years. Her previous experience has encompassed a wide range of research and educational activities and she has been involved in promoting career development for many years. She is currently a part-time GP, Head of the Stoke-on-Trent Teaching Primary Care Trust programme, and clinical dean at Staffordshire University. Ruth has researched and written about the need for careers support services in the NHS and run career guidance skills training around the UK. She ran a support scheme for doctors and dentists in Staffordshire for nearly ten years, with career counselling as a component resource. One of her most formative experiences was an in-depth career review that led to her diversifying within an academic/clinical career.

Wendy Garcarz is an education and development specialist with a proven record of accomplishment in primary care. She has 20 years' experience in education and training management in both the public and private sectors. She has spent the last ten years working in primary care, developing primary care clinicians and support workers in service commissioning, continuing professional development, strategic planning and service innovations. Wendy is the Chief Executive of 4-health, an organisational development consultancy specialising in sustainable change through workforce investment. She and her colleagues work with all types of healthcare organisations. wendy@4-health.biz.

Neil Houston left school intending to become an accountant, but before setting foot in an office changed course and applied to study medicine. He now works half-time as a GP in a rural practice in central Scotland. He has a number of educational and quality improvement roles and works with primary care teams as an associate adviser in professional development. He has recently been involved in developing and evaluating a career guidance programme for primary healthcare professionals.

Anne Longbottom began her working life in a bank in Birmingham where she quickly progressed to working with managers in assessing individual and corporate lending proposals. Following a career break to bring up her son, she rejoined the jobs market in a local primary school and began working in a local further education college in the Faculty of Caring Services. Here she gained a valuable insight into working in care settings. Her desire to ensure that all staff within an organisation had the opportunity to develop and progress began to flourish. Anne now works within the NHS to promote learning and development for staff who traditionally have found it more difficult to access training opportunities. Anne is an active member of the Guide Association and a mentor for new leaders.

Kay Mohanna has made several changes in her life and career without the benefit of objective careers advice or guidance. She undertook research as the Royal College of General Practitioners' Midland Faculty young practitioners' fellow in 1997–98 to reveal the need for career support for GPs in the early years of practice, producing a resource booklet as an output of her post. During her academic career as a Principal Lecturer in Medical Education at Staffordshire University, Kay has met and helped many doctors with their career development. Their experiences illustrate their need for interested careers advisers with objective and up-to-date information about alternative career pathways. Kay has co-authored a book with Ruth about medical career guidance, and run national seminars for doctors aiding their career decisions.

Fiona Taylor spent 20 years as a GP then psychiatrist, and now runs a career consultancy with a special interest in doctors' careers. Her professional and personal life has tended to be colourful from an upbringing among one of Africa's most primitive tribes, being GP to the homeless, repeatedly acting as hostess to the royal family, to working as psychiatrist to the criminally insane. Her main interest is in helping people create or move into jobs that suit them. These are jobs where they will perform well and be motivated and satisfied. fiona@calm.uk.com.

Acknowledgements

The careers information in the Appendices was collated as part of a service development project commissioned by the Workforce Development Directorate of Shropshire and Staffordshire Health Authority from a team at Staffordshire University. We thank Shelagh Cobb for her hard work in collecting this information for health professionals and managers working in primary care.

Glossary of terms

Career counselling: is an umbrella term for the process of enabling somebody to evaluate their current situation and identify what steps are needed in order to change. It will usually include identification of a person's strengths and weaknesses in relation to work options and may also include careers information.[1]

Careers guidance: is personal and directive, and provides *advice* within the context of the opportunities that are available.[1]

Careers information: covers the facts about the qualifications and experience needed for alternative career pathways and the opportunities that there are for career progression. That is, the number and type of posts available at a particular level and in a particular specialty, and details of the qualifications and training necessary.[1]

Coaching: is the process of motivating, encouraging and helping an individual to improve their skills, knowledge and attitudes in a framework of goal setting and achievement.[2]

Mentoring: is the process whereby an experienced, highly regarded empathic person (the mentor) guides another individual (the mentee) in the development and re-examination of their own ideas, learning and personal and professional development.[3]

Reflection: is the process whereby people actively deliberate on their performance or the care they deliver and identify their strengths and weaknesses (as individuals or in groups).

Skills escalator: is an approach to developing careers in the NHS through a supportive culture and infrastructure. The vision of a modernised NHS is for staff to have a range of options for developing and extending their careers, supported by learning and development opportunities. Getting people on the escalator means attracting a wide range of people to work within the NHS by offering advice and help and a variety of career and training step-on and step-off points. Enabling staff to move on the escalator is about encouraging staff to renew and extend their skills and knowledge to gain stimulating careers through a strategy of lifelong learning.[4]

References

1 Chambers R, Mohanna K and Field S (2000) *Opportunities and Options in Medical Careers.* Radcliffe Medical Press, Oxford.

2 Chambers R, Mohanna K, Wakley G and Wall D (2004) *Demonstrating Your Competence 1. Healthcare teaching.* Radcliffe Medical Press, Oxford.

3 Standing Committee on Postgraduate Medical and Dental Education (1998) *An Enquiry into Mentoring; supporting doctors and dentists at work.* Standing Committee on Postgraduate Medical and Dental Education, London.

4 Department of Health (2004) *Skills Escalator. Achieving your potential.* Department of Health, London.

Introduction

You wouldn't be reading this book unless you were wondering if there is anything you can do to enhance or change your career. You may just be seeking reassurance that you are reasonably content in your current job, or alternatively wanting to review your whole career, feeling that working in the NHS is not for you. You might just want to check out what other opportunities there are for your future career. You could be finding that the other pressures in your life in combination with a busy job in the NHS are just too much. More flexible working hours might help you cope with looking after young children or elderly dependants, or struggle with physical or mental ill-health, or other unsettling personal events.

The material in this book has evolved to help people like you plan their careers in the NHS. What you learn could help you to enable colleagues to plan and develop their careers too, if that is part of your work role and responsibilities as line manager or tutor or appraiser.

We need to recruit and retain additional doctors, other independent contractors such as dentists, pharmacists, optometrists, nurses, allied health professionals, managers and other staff. NHS staff with low morale may opt for early retirement or part-time working. The challenge for the NHS is to create a working environment that encourages you and your colleagues to stay working as long as possible. The expertise of managers and others may be lost in NHS reorganisations where there are no obvious alternative career pathways, and support for career development is inadequate.

As each NHS reorganisation and innovation occurs with newly created opportunities for health professionals in leadership and management, there is an incipient drain of the health professional workforce away from their clinical posts. New clinically based career opportunities have sprung up with the shift to more community-based working for hospital consultants and nurses, and more specialist roles for general practitioners (GPs), nurses and allied health professionals with special interests. Information about these opportunities is not easily available to all.

Many health professionals undergo multiple transitions during their career pathways. Yet there is little known about the sources of careers information they access, and limited availability of good careers guidance, support and advice services.[1] Health professionals and managers may be in posts to which they are ill suited. They may have pursued different career pathways if appropriate careers advice had been readily available earlier on, and throughout their careers. And for many, their career objectives and career progress is central to their personal morale and job satisfaction.[2,3]

Career planning

Career planning is a must at all stages of a health service career, for students or young professionals uncertain of their career paths, for established clinicians faced with a range of career opportunities and dilemmas, or when thinking of retirement. A first step is to learn more about yourself. To discover your personal strengths, career and job preferences, motivation and priorities in life, you should know how you want to balance the time you spend between work and leisure, and between time and effort of work and income. You should understand what levels of responsibility, challenge and interaction with other people suit your personal style.[4,5]

Your career plans may centre on developing your particular skills and interests within the specialty in which you are working so that you function more effectively. You may want to develop your career so that you become more specialised in a particular clinical or managerial area. You might want more variety in your work and decide to develop a parallel area of interest or a new skill that enhances your current post. It may be promotion that you are after with more status or responsibility. You may crave a complete change – in a new career that is a natural extension of your current work, or as a fresh start in a different career within or outside the health service.

There are gender differences in the way that clinicians choose their clinical specialty, the likelihood of progressing to senior positions and the proportions who work less than full-time. Male doctors, for instance, are more likely to choose their specialties based on 'interest in the specialty', 'promotion' and 'financial prospects'. Women more often choose 'close contact with patients', 'a job in the right geographical area', 'fitting in with family life' and 'availability of part-time work' as important features of their selected career specialties.[6]

Career challenge

Everyone should take stock and review their options throughout their careers. Various triggers might occur in your life that prompt you to ask yourself whether you are happy at work, whether you are in the right job and whether it is worth rethinking your present career, such as when:

- you are faced with a variety of opportunities and options, uncertain of which career path to take
- you feel there is a mismatch between you and your particular career – maybe your personal ethics or values are threatened, or your needs and preferences have changed
- you feel demotivated or dissatisfied with your work – maybe your role has changed, or you feel your career has plateaued for too long
- a serious life event occurs – bereavement, getting married, going through a divorce, developing an illness or disability
- a significant event occurs at work – a complaint from a patient, the traumatic death of a patient, you making a mistake, a critical incident arising from work such as you or a colleague being subject to a dispute or personal attack
- you are preparing for retirement – wanting to slow down but not stop.

Your career will be more satisfying and rewarding if you can be flexible and adaptable in the face of the changes and surprises that life will inevitably throw at you. These changes might be personal circumstances (such as illness or starting a family) or external ones (such as changes in training or working hours).[7]

References

1 Chambers R, Cobb S, Mohanna K *et al.* (2003) *Improving the Quality of Careers Information and Guidance in Primary Care*. Staffordshire University, Stafford.
2 Mercer G (1979) *The Employment of Nurses*. Croom Helm, London.
3 Mackay L (1989) Career women. *Nurs Times.* **84:** 42–4.

4 Kent S (1997) *Creating your own Career. Practical advice for graduates in a changing world.* Kogan Page, London.

5 Leider R (1994) *Life Skills; Taking Charge of your Personal and Professional Growth.* Pfeiffer and Company, London.

6 Baldwin P (1999) Cohort studies of Scottish medical school graduates. In: *First Oxford Conference on Medical Careers.* Oxford University, Oxford.

7 MacDonald R (2003) *My Beautiful Career.* BMJ careers workbook. BMJcareers, London. bmjcareers.com

1

Career planning is a must for you

Wendy Garcarz and Ruth Chambers

Career planning is the process you will go through to actively manage your career, consider your personal development needs, and decide how best you can access development opportunities. It helps you to identify the factors that are important to you in your chosen profession and build up a picture of your priorities in terms of skills, interests and what motivates you. People who have been in the same role for a while can reassess their career to date and recognise new opportunities, gaps in their knowledge or skills or experience and consider how they can meet these.

Make career planning work for you

Our tips for managing your career are:

- consider what you want or need from your career and what you can offer in return
- recognise your transferable skills and the competencies you have already developed over time
- develop one or more career goals
- be flexible about change so that you can take advantage of opportunities as they crop up
- promote an accurate profile of yourself: maximise your strengths, acknowledge your weaknesses or inexperience and what you are doing to address these
- understand the value of your contribution to others and their work programmes in various health settings or organisations
- plan for your future – never stop – even if it is to get ready for a fulfilling retirement.

Consider the changing world of work in the NHS in relation to the planning and review of your career. Your career planning needs to be done in the context of the professional climate and likely changes to the way the health service is organised and changing. For instance the current emphasis on flexible working practices means that you can combine more than one post into a portfolio career (*see* Chapter 6 for more on this). New information and communication technologies make it easier to work from home or travel less using email, web cams, telephone and videoconferencing etc. New technologies in the health service require people with different skills to operate them or deliver the redesigned service. Secondment opportunities are more commonplace and varied, as some short-term posts are set up to introduce the changes.

Clinical professionals working for the NHS have traditionally had predictable career pathways with clear boundaries that did not provide the flexibility or opportunity desired by many. But the need for the NHS to retain an ageing workforce has meant that employers are looking for ways to adapt jobs to match the needs or preferences of individual members of staff. A learning culture is being evolved in many trusts where professional development is valued and investments made in training and supporting staff whatever their discipline or seniority, to acquire new skills and competencies, so that they gain new qualifications and experience at all stages in their careers.

People can have more than one career in their working lifespan (although it may be in the same field such as combining being a clinician, medical author and health economist) and these changes and variety can be motivational and fulfilling.

Your healthy career

The word *career* sometimes has negative connotations related to ambition, overwork, poor work/life balance, stress and unhealthy competition. But *career* simply means a series of jobs in a profession or occupation that an individual has throughout their life. It should be about the balance between an individual's work and their personal life and reflect their aspirations, beliefs and values. So your career should be a positive driving force in your life rather than the negative or nuisance part that gets in the way of the rest of your life (*see* Box 1.1).

Box 1.1:   Checklist for a healthy career

- What do I *want* to do?
- What *can* I do?
- What am I *going* to do?

Factors to consider in choosing a career specialty or interest

When reviewing your current job or weighing up the potential for a career move, you should consider the match between you and the job as to whether:

- you have the sort of personality that fits with the requirements of the job
- you have the appropriate skills, training and experience
- you have sufficient job satisfaction and interest in your work
- you are sufficiently motivated to work effectively
- the job fits with your ethics, inner values and boundaries
- the job provides the balance you want between work and your off-duty life.

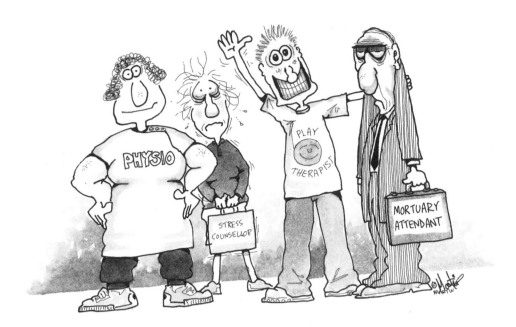

Develop one or more career goals

Having a clear idea about the direction of your career gives you the elements of choice and control. You need that overall vision. How will you know if you have achieved your career goal if you do not have a vision for the future? Identify what you are aiming for and the nature of the milestones that will describe how you are going to get there. This does not mean that you cannot change your career plan if your circumstances should change; it is essential to your success to be flexible.

Lifelong learning

You need to learn new skills, take on new knowledge, develop new behaviours and attitudes throughout your life to keep pace with life's changes. Sorry, that basic qualification will not see you through your career these days without continuing to learn more and more ... you should always be open to the next challenge. Learning should help you to relish change as it means that you will learn something new and develop as a result.

Postgraduate educational qualifications can be fitted around your regular job if you can arrange study time or opt for work-based learning. Assignments can be built into your current role and responsibilities and give added value to your practice or trust, so that you can negotiate protected time to undertake it.

Everyone working for the NHS should set out a personal educational development plan that they review each year as part of the appraisal process. Career development should be an integral part of such a plan, setting out goals for the forthcoming year and beyond, and describing realistic ways of achieving those career goals.

You cannot consider your own individual needs and plans in isolation from those of the rest of your work team or organisation, or the needs of the NHS as a whole. There needs to be an opening for such a post or the new skills you intend to develop. A successful personal development plan (PDP) must balance competing influences and pressures of service needs and NHS priorities while enabling individual staff to *stay in control* of the development of their careers and working lives and retain their organisation's and colleagues' support.

Job evaluation

The NHS job evaluation scheme helps to make sure that staff are rewarded fairly; and ensures that the NHS respects the principles of equal pay for work of equal value.[1] *See* Chapter 5 for more details.

Job satisfaction and career fulfilment

Job satisfaction is known to protect you from the effects of stress from work. So increasing your job satisfaction is one of the best ways to 'stress proof' yourself against the pressures and demands of a job. You will minimise the effects of the elements of the job you find more stressful if you enjoy your job, feel valued and are in control of your everyday work. Low job satisfaction can affect your performance at work – one example is the link between low job satisfaction and poor prescribing practice.[2,3]

Motivation

People are motivated by different things. Money, fame, power are all key motivators. Pride, lust, anger, gluttony, envy, sloth and covetousness are all listed as prime motivators – hopefully not all of these are relevant to any great extent for you working in the NHS! Some of the best motivators for fulfilling your needs are:

- interesting and/or useful work
- sense of achievement
- responsibility
- opportunities for career progression or professional development
- gaining new skills or competencies
- sense of belonging to a directorate or practice team or the NHS.

Maslow's hierarchy of a person's needs describes how self-esteem and fulfilment are not possible if the basic structure and safety components of their life are insecure.[4]

Fulfilment and personal growth are only likely to occur if the basics of an individual's life are in place. Self-esteem, status and recognition from others are only possible if they are built upon a good social base that includes love, friendship, belonging to groups (work, home, leisure, professional), and social activities. Fulfilment, maturity and wisdom are only possible where all the other conditions encourage growth, personal development and accomplishment. If you are contemplating a career change or expansion of your career that will require new skills, knowledge and experiences, you might be better waiting until your personal life is reasonably settled and you feel secure, before making major alterations or moving on.

Transferable skills and competencies

In a fast-paced environment like the NHS where change is a common facet of your working life, professional requirements evolve continually and you will be expected to be flexible and move with the times. So you should capitalise on your skills. Recognise your strengths, personal attributes and experiences (whatever the source, maybe from outside the NHS), and transfer those into your everyday work, applying them to the next task or challenge that presents itself. Try to get a more objective view of your performance and development needs, with input from other people or by comparing outcomes of your work against the standards of best practice expected of you.

Quality and standards

You will also be working to the quality standards set by your practice or trust or the NHS in general, as well as personal standards that you as a health professional or manager work to. Aiming for quality is a prerequisite to a healthy career, as it forms the basic measurement for your achievement and reward – practical and intrinsic satisfaction. Make sure that it is obvious what your contribution is to organisational success, as well as taking satisfaction from the difference you make to patient care as an individual.

Create an impression

If you are keen to develop your career, recognise that you may be employable by a number of organisations within or outside the NHS. Think what it is that makes you marketable. Find ways to raise your profile so that you are considered for exciting projects or developmental work when they crop up.[5] You need to become an effective self-publicist and communicate your successes to the right people. Do not rest on your laurels and wait to be discovered. This kind of self-publicity may not sit easily with you. Many people are shy of pushing themselves forward or seeking credit for work they have done well. But if you do not take that credit visibly, someone else will – who does not deserve it. The world's a tough place.

Networking

Networking is the life blood of career development. A next career move is often dependent on your relations with your peers or colleagues, managers and professional contacts. These other people are a valuable source of information and resources. They can offer sources of expertise or connections, and mixing with them can be a breeding ground for sharing good practice. Much of networking is of mutual benefit to both parties – they need you and your ideas or support as much as you need theirs. This is where your future referees may be drawn from, or people who push you forward for promotion or other opportunities.[6]

Become recognised for making change happen

All organisations need effective ways of managing change and for most (on a practical level), that means managing people through change. The skills required are generic communications and people management based. Becoming such a change agent in an organisation involves you in flexible working, motivational skills, changing roles, uncertain job titles, short-term assignments and the ability to inspire others beyond their anxieties. These types of individuals are rare but incredibly valuable to an organisation, as they are the only type of people that can deliver sustainable change in that organisation, by finding ways to overcome the barriers to change and taking people along with them.[5,7]

Plan for your future

Formulating your personal aspirations and defining career opportunities are essential for career planning. People need to be at least one step ahead of their career development, and this forward planning should be evident in actions, such as working to gain qualifications that will fit you for the future posts you envisage. If you do not underpin your career aspirations by cultivating the right networks or gaining new skills or qualifications then your career plan is likely to remain just that – a plan!

Reflect on what you are looking for from your work:

- the kind of work you enjoy – routine, exciting, prestigious, quiet and steady
- the setting in which you want to work – community, hospital, rural, urban, travel
- the type of people for whom you want to care – the ages and characteristics of patients
- the type of people with whom you want to work – and whether in a small team or big organisation
- the extent of patient contact that suits you
- the level of income you consider (i) essential and (ii) desirable
- the working hours, holidays, study leave: how the hours fit with your current state and future domestic plans
- opportunities for parallel career interests such as research, writing, education, consultancy, private work or work-related hobbies
- the extent of professional autonomy and responsibility you want.

You will also need to take account of:

- the details of any training required – hours, practical difficulties, examinations
- the job prospects of alternative career paths: the opportunities for you to progress, or the competition ratio – that is, the number of people trying to get a more senior job in a particular area relative to the number of senior posts that exist.

It's rewarding but very difficult, involving compromise and sacrifice of family life.[6]

Self-sufficiency

You need to develop some degree of self-sufficiency as a vital component in your healthy career. At times, you need to be able to operate effectively in the absence of external recognition or praise, without receiving any feedback or direction and even so maintain a realistic outlook that is upbeat. Optimism and pessimism are both contagious. You want your practice or trust to consider you as an asset, not someone who is part of the problem but part of the solution. So the knack is to maintain this optimistic and positive persona even if no one is telling you how well you are doing.

Invest in yourself

In the breakneck speed of working life it is difficult to find the time or energy to invest in yourself. Reflective practice is about reviewing your experiences and considering your development needs. You need protected thinking time. Just as time spent considering project outcomes and what might be done differently can improve future results significantly, you can reflect on your career progress, but that takes time. Reflection just has to be carried out consistently (for example one hour spread over a month) and does not have to take up days or weeks. Turn to Chapter 2 for a whole series of reflective exercises you can do in relation to evaluating and planning your career.

Leadership

Leaders can and do emerge from all areas and levels in the health service. Leadership works well when it is of a shared and collaborative nature in a practice or trust, and is not just the sole responsibility of senior staff. As a leader you will become aware that a change is necessary, visualise how change could make an improvement and help lead others along the path of change until it becomes the new 'normal' state.[7]

Life/work balance

Pursuing a fulfilling career should be about working smarter rather than working harder. The work/life balance is now as important to some individuals as any financial rewards. Working longer hours will not necessarily help you to work more effectively. Many people experience a tension between work and home demands, and it is difficult to juggle home and work priorities and set time aside to keep fit and relax. But you must try to achieve a good balance to give you an intellectual edge and help you to maintain your sense of perspective. It requires self-discipline to set personal boundaries, self-confidence to view your time as equally important to that of other people, and energy to redesign your daily habits. Career health is dependent on your physical and mental wellbeing and retaining a sense of proportion in terms of what is really important in life. Your career is just one element of your life, so do get it in perspective.

> If I had worked full-time I never would have seen my husband and childcare was impossible where we lived. Now I could do full-time I don't want to – too old!![6]

There are no hard and fast rules about how much time you should spend on work-related activities compared to the rest of your life. Sensible advice is to divide your day as:[8]

- 45–55% on personal needs (including sleeping, chores, basic care)
- 25–30% on work
- 20–25% on leisure.

Only you and your partner at home know if you are getting the balance right. And if you have not got a 'partner at home' to discuss the balance with, maybe it's time you reduced your wholesale commitment to work and socialised more. If you increase the proportion of work, it is the leisure component that is reduced proportionately.

The impact of your career on those at home

Do not forget the impact of your career choice upon your partner and family at home – if that is relevant to your own circumstances. Your family may not be tolerant of you prioritising your career, or studying for further qualifications or making a house move to take up a different post.

> My social circumstances – mother of two small children, working part-time – influence my career decisions far more than availability or otherwise of careers information.[9]

The 'psychological contract' between you and your boss

The psychological contract between employer and employee is slowly disappearing in the UK. Employees could expect some degree of security and certainty about their jobs in return for loyalty and employers that recognised and valued their past and future contributions. On the whole, job security can no longer be guaranteed and, in general, employers need to ensure commitment and high performance of individuals by creating a different kind of 'psychological contract'. Consider your understanding of what your organisation wants. This could be for example the competencies and level of performance they require of you, as well as your management style. Then negotiate what you can offer in return for what you want from your organisation. This could include job satisfaction, high salary, flexible working, good working conditions and environment, and opportunities for career development. Ideally this should be a two-way process with both the employee and employer feeling that they are getting something out of their working relationship.

Career catastrophe[10]

A career catastrophe could be anything that abruptly alters the way you think about your career path. The factors that might temporarily or permanently derail your career can be divided into internal and external factors, and some are listed in Box 1.2. You may have your own additions. You might consider one or more career catastrophe(s) now because it has recently happened to you or because you are planning ahead in case it does. One example of a career catastrophe might be you developing a physical or mental impairment that interferes with your work sufficiently for it to be difficult for you to continue in your post, or that might even put patient safety at risk. In that case you will have no choice but to stop and revise your role and responsibilities within your specialty area or change career to another clinical or non-clinical position.

Box 1.2: Examples of factors that may affect the smooth flow of your career pathway

Internal factors

- Illness e.g. short-term such as fractured limb; long-term such as depression or chronic condition
- Burnout
- Job dissatisfaction
- Change of priorities, including positive changes
- Pregnancy
- Mismatch with intended career – personality, skills

External factors

- Lack of career progression, lack of jobs
- Complaints
- Immigration rules
- Trust reconfiguration/enforced redundancy
- Discrimination (age, gender, race, disability)
- 'The establishment' – 'old boy network'
- Family's competing needs – housing, education, income, family illness
- Personal circumstances change e.g. divorce, bereavement

Career anchors

Appreciating your personal ethics and work values in any career

Integral to the process of career planning is having a real understanding of yourself; what motivates and what inspires you and what does not. Your life experiences, your principles and values, your relationships with family, friends and colleagues and professional identity influence your career choices. Therefore, the greater your self-awareness the more satisfying your career choices could be.

Your ethics set the boundaries as to how far you are prepared to go to get what you want. Work values are personal to you too. You will be happiest and most fulfilled in a job that incorporates your main work values. Eight career anchor categories have been identified by Schein to increase people's insights into their strengths and motivation as part of career development. These are:

- technical or functional competence
- general managerial competence
- autonomy or independence
- security or stability
- entrepreneurial creativity
- service or dedication to a cause
- pure challenge
- lifestyle.[11]

People define their self-image in terms of these traits and come to understand more about their talents, motives and values – and which of these they would not give up if forced to make a choice.

Career anchors help you to understand the meaning and implications of past career decisions and inform future ones, whether or not you work in the health service. They give a clearer understanding of:

- your orientations towards work
- your motives
- your values
- your talents.

Career anchors will help you to:

- define the themes and patterns that are dominant in your life
- understand your own approach to your work and career
- identify and clarify your talents
- provide reasons for career choices
- take action to secure a fulfilling career.

The questions listed in Table 1.1 will help you to identify your career anchors and prompt you to consider your areas of competence, values and motivation. Read through the detailed descriptions that follow and then come back to complete the box. Fill in the middle column, rating how important you perceive each career anchor to be for you. Then complete the right-hand column, gauging how you rate each career anchor in respect of the main job you currently hold. Add another column or two if you have a portfolio of other jobs and you want to think about each one individually with a separate column for each.

Table 1.1: Identify your career anchors and how well you perceive these to match your current job

Schein career anchor[11]	How important is this aspect of your career to you (score out of 5 where 0 is nil and 5 is a great deal)?	How does this match with your current situation (score out of 5 where 0 is nil and 5 is a great deal)?
Technical or functional competence		
Managerial competence		
Autonomy or independence		
Security or stability		
Entrepreneurial or creative		
Service or dedication to a cause		
Pure challenge		
Lifestyle		

Is there a mismatch between what career anchors you rate as being most important for you and those that relate to your current situation?

Career anchor descriptions

Technical and functional competence

A high score in this area suggests that you value being able to apply your skills and to develop those skills to an ever higher level. You derive your sense of identity from the exercise of your skills and are happiest when your work permits you to be challenged in these skilled areas. You may be willing to manage others in your technical or functional area, but you are not interested in management for its own sake, and would avoid general management because you would have to move away from your own area of expertise.

General managerial competence

A high score in this area suggests that you value the opportunity to climb to a high enough level to enable you to integrate the efforts of others across functions and to be responsible for the output of a particular unit in your trust or practice, or other organisation. You want to be responsible and accountable for total results, and you identify your own work with the success of the organisation for which you work. If you are presently in a technical or functional area, you view that as a necessary learning experience; however, your ambition is to get to a generalist job as soon as possible. Being at a high managerial level in a specialist function does not interest you.

Autonomy and independence

A high score in this area suggests that you value the opportunity to define your own work in your own way. You want to remain in jobs that allow you flexibility regarding how and when you work. If you tend to dislike organisational rules and restrictions to any degree, you are attracted to occupations with the freedom you seek, such as teaching or consulting. You may turn down opportunities for promotion or advancement in order to retain autonomy. You may opt to set up and run a business of your own in order to achieve a sense of autonomy; however, this motive is not the same as entrepreneurial creativity described below.

Security and stability

A high score in this area suggests that you value employment security or tenure in a job or organisation. This career anchor reveals your concern for financial security (such as pension and retirement plans) or employment security. Such longed for stability may involve trading your loyalty and willingness to do whatever your employer wants, for some promise of job tenure. You are less concerned with the content of your work and the rank you achieve in the organisation, although you may achieve a high level if your talents permit. As with autonomy, everyone has certain needs for security and stability, especially at times when financial burdens may be heavy (that mortgage or those school fees) or when you are facing retirement. But people anchored in this way are *always* concerned with these issues and build their entire self-image around security and stability.

Entrepreneurial creativity

A high score in this area suggests that you value the opportunity to create an organisation or enterprise of your own, built on your own abilities and your willingness to take risks and to overcome obstacles. You want to prove that you can create an enterprise that is the result of your own efforts. You may be working for others in an organisation while you are learning and assessing future opportunities, but you may go out on your own as soon as you feel you can manage it. You will want your enterprise to be financially successful as proof of your abilities.

Service and dedication to a cause

A high score in this area suggests that you value being able to pursue work that achieves something, such as making the world a better place to live, solving environmental problems, improving harmony among people, helping others, improving people's safety, curing diseases through new products, and so on. You pursue such opportunities even if it means changing organisations, and you do not accept transfers or promotions that would take you out of work that fulfils those values.

Pure challenge

A high score in this area suggests that you value the opportunity to work on solutions to seemingly unsolvable problems, to win out over tough opponents, or to overcome difficult obstacles. For you, the only meaningful reason for pursuing a job or career is that it permits you to achieve the impossible. Some people find such pure challenge in intellectual kinds of work, such as the engineer who is only interested in impossibly difficult designs; some find the challenge in complex multifaceted situations such as the strategy consultant who is only interested in clients who are about to go bankrupt and have exhausted all other resources; some find it in interpersonal competition such as the professional athlete. Novelty, variety, and difficulty become ends in themselves, and if something is easy it becomes immediately boring.

> It's not an easy career [medicine]. Decide if you are really determined, think long and hard. Lots of time has to be committed but it is rewarding at the end.[6]

Lifestyle

A high score in this area suggests that you value being able to balance and integrate your personal needs, family needs and the requirements of your career. You want to bring all the major sectors of your life and work together towards an integrated whole. So you need a career situation that is flexible enough to achieve such integration. You may have to sacrifice some aspects of your career (for example, refuse a geographical move that would be a promotion that would upset your total life situation), and you define your achievements in broader terms than just career successes. Identity is more tied up with how you live your total life, where you settle, how you deal with your family situation and how you develop yourself, than with any particular job or organisation.

> Go for it – and consider working less than full-time or diversifying in order to recharge your batteries, even if it means earning a bit less.[6]

Discover your hidden talents

Make time for career planning. Take stock and review your career to date. Evaluate your strengths and skills and decide what you want to do, to continue in your current path or diversify to parallel or alternative fields. Then, taking account of the opportunities on offer and any circumstances limiting your choice of actions, push on with your career development and achieve your career goals.[12,13]

Activity 1.1:   The challenge is to create your vision for your beautiful career[14]

So where are you now?

What are you proud of in your personal life and job?

What can you celebrate?

What would you like to be different?

References

1   Department of Health (2004) *NHS Job Evaluation Handbook* (2e). Department of Health, London. www.dh.gov.uk/assetRoot/04/09/37/39/04093739.pdf

2   Sutherland V and Cooper C (1993) Identifying distress among general practitioners: predictors of psychological ill-health and job dissatisfaction. *Soc Sci Med.* **37:** 575–81.

3   Ramirez A, Graham J, Richards M *et al.* (1996) Mental health of hospital consultants: the effects of stress and satisfaction at work. *Lancet.* **347:** 724–8.

4   Maslow AH (1970) *Motivation and Personality.* Harper and Row, New York.

5   Lilley R and Bowden G (2000) *Managing the Message. A toolkit for health service communicators.* Radcliffe Medical Press, Oxford.

6   Chambers R, Mohanna K and Chambers S (2003) *Survival Skills for Doctors and their Families.* Radcliffe Medical Press, Oxford.

7   Martin V (2003) *Leading Change in Health and Social Care.* Routledge, London.

8   Chambers R (1999) *Survival Skills for GPs.* Radcliffe Medical Press, Oxford.

9   Chambers R, Cobb S, Mohanna K *et al.* (2003) *Improving the Quality of Careers Information and Guidance in Primary Care.* Staffordshire University, Stafford.

10 Mohanna K and Chambers R (2003) Career crises. *BMJ Career Focus.* **326:** s35–6.

11 Schein E (1996) *Career Anchors, Discovering your Real Values.* Pfeiffer, Oxford.

12 Learndirect (2003) *Discover your Hidden Talents.* The Open University, Milton Keynes. www.learndirect-advice.co.uk

13 Langdon K (2004) *Cultivate a Cool Career.* Infinite Ideas, Oxford.

14 MacDonald R (2003) *My Beautiful Career.* BMJ careers workbook. BMJcareers, London. bmjcareers.com

2

The nuts and bolts of career planning: a practical guide

Fiona Taylor and Neil Houston

Forty per cent of you at any one time will be questioning your career. This takes the form of 'Why on earth am I doing this?!' – on a bad day. But at other calmer moments you might try and look at your career in a more dispassionate and reflective way. Even then it can be impossible to know where to start. In general, we are not good at identifying either our own skills and potential or the career opportunities that exist for us out there.

This chapter offers you a structure around which to start to review and plan your career development. It takes the form of a series of exercises, which you can do individually or with the help of someone who knows you well. They will give you more insight into your strengths and preferences and how well these match your current career, then help you to focus on how you want your career to develop. Careers can only do two things; they either develop or stagnate. Which is yours doing at the present time?

We pose three challenges through the exercises in this chapter:

- where are you now?
- where do you want to be?
- how are you going to get there?

Where are you now?

It is worth looking at why you ended up in a particular area of work and why you continue to work in that field. The reasons are often strikingly different. Look at the example in the case study and see how Angela became stuck in a career rut.

Case study 2.1: Example of a career rut

Angela Crossman is a 30-year-old practice nurse. As a teenager she wanted to become a nurse because she admired her glamorous aunt who was a nurse. With hindsight she realises the glamour was because the aunt lived in Australia and worked with the flying doctor service. She is still working as a nurse because she enjoys the contact with people, shares the financial burden of bringing up a young family with her partner and cannot think what else she would do.

Now it is your turn. Have a go at answering the two core questions in Activity 2.1 and then Activity 2.2.

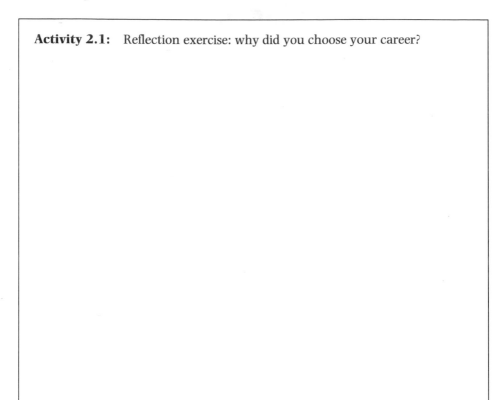

Activity 2.1:   Reflection exercise: why did you choose your career?

Activity 2.2:   Reflection exercise: why are you still working in this career or area?

How did it go? Did you find that the reasons you entered your current specialty or career still featured as reasons why you are working in it today? Or have you lost sight of the original reasons for entering your career or taking up your particular post? There may be even more reasons for you continuing to work there than there were originally of course.

What can you give to a job? What do you need from your job?

One way of thinking about your job is captured in Figure 2.1 in terms of what you:

- give to your job e.g. your skills, experience, real interest, energy and time
- need from your job e.g. motivation, money, work/life balance, security, challenge.

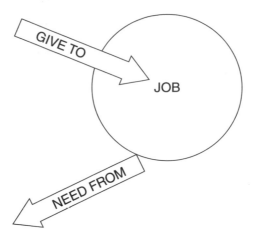

Figure 2.1:   What you give to and need from a job.

Now it is your turn to reflect on your career again. Complete Activity 2.3, thinking of your *career in general*.

Activity 2.3:   Reflection exercise: what can you give to your career and what do you need from it?

What can you give to a job?   What do you need from your job?

Now compare this general perspective in Activity 2.3 with what your *current* post is giving you by completing Activity 2.4.

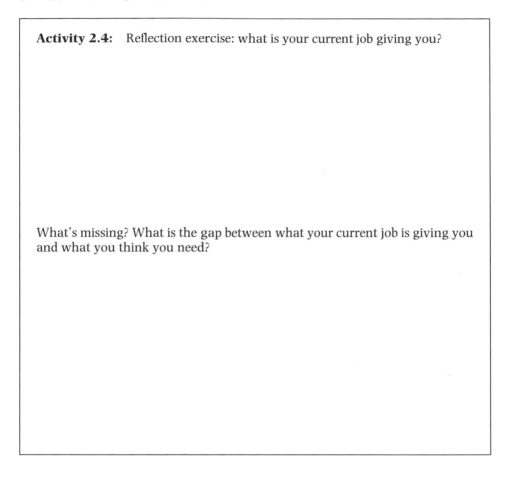

Activity 2.4:   Reflection exercise: what is your current job giving you?

What's missing? What is the gap between what your current job is giving you and what you think you need?

What are your skills?

Your skills are often the reason you were appointed to a particular position. Individuals however have great difficulty identifying the generic skills they possess, and tend to concentrate on the traditional skills of their profession such as clinical or organisational ones. But you actually have a multitude of skills.

The following exercise that runs from Activities 2.5 to 2.9 is designed to help you to identify the skills you possess and profile the ones you would like to develop further. The skills are arranged into five categories:

- people skills
- skills in handling information
- practical skills
- analytical skills
- specialist skills e.g. the ability to read an X-ray accurately, or diagnose complex cases in a particular clinical field.

Look through the list in each of Activities 2.5, 2.6, 2.7, 2.8 and 2.9 and identify the skills you feel you possess by writing *yes* or *no* in the appropriate column for each row. You could ask a colleague to go through the list commenting on whether you have those skills, as well. You will often find that you have skills that you use all the time of which you are unaware, but which your colleagues recognise.

Activity 2.5:   Reflection exercise: check out your people skills

People skill	*Already have the skill*	*Want to develop the skill*
Advising		
Assessing		
Communicating (oral)		
Communicating (written)		
Controlling		
Counselling		
Decision making		
Delegating		
Developing rapport		
Directing		
Facilitating		
Guiding		
Initiating		
Leading		
Managing		
Managing conflict		
Mentoring		
Motivating		
Negotiating		
Organising		
Performing		
Persuading		
Presenting		
Recruiting		
Serving		
Sharing		
Supervising		
Taking responsibility		
Teaching		
Training		
Using intuition		

Activity 2.6: Reflection exercise: check out your skills in handling information

Skill in handling information	Already have the skill	Want to develop the skill
Administering		
Arranging information		
Budgeting		
Compiling		
Computing		
Editing		
Evaluating		
Marketing		
Organising		
Presenting		
Reading		
Simplifying		
Translating		

Activity 2.7: Reflection exercise: check out your practical skills

Practical skill	Already have the skill	Want to develop the skill
Arranging		
Assembling		
Building		
Co-ordination		
Creating		
Demonstrating		
Designing		
Improving		
Inspecting		
Installing		
Inventing		
Making		
Operating		
Repairing		
Testing		

Activity 2.8:   Reflection exercise: check out your analytical skills

Analytical skill	Already have the skill	Want to develop the skill
Analysing		
Assessing		
Auditing		
Communicating (written)		
Creating		
Debating		
Deciding		
Developing		
Diagnosing		
Evaluating		
Expanding		
Experimenting		
Identifying opportunities		
Identifying priorities		
Innovating		
Instructing		
Interpreting		
Learning		
Memorising		
Observing		
Organising		
Planning		
Problem solving		
Reporting		
Researching		
Resolving		
Shaping		
Simplifying		
Using numbers		

Activity 2.9:   Reflection exercise: check out your specialist skills

Specialist skill (add skills relevant to your specialism)	*Already have the skill*	*Want to develop the skill*

If you had to pick out your top three skills, which would they be? Describe them in the following activity.

Activity 2.10:   Which three skills are you especially good at and do you enjoy using?

Did you come across or think of any skills that you would like to develop further? Make a note of them now to include in your career development plan later on.

What do you do well and enjoy?

You have identified what you are good at. Now how about identifying the things that you do not do so well. This can be easier than identifying your skills! Work through these next four activities thinking of things you do both inside and outside of work. Ask a colleague or member of your family to verify that you have produced a complete and accurate list in relation to work or outside work for your answers to Activities 2.11 to 2.15.

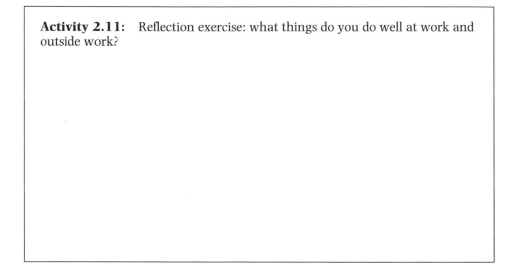

Activity 2.11:   Reflection exercise: what things do you do well at work and outside work?

Activity 2.12:   Reflection exercise: what things do you do badly at work and outside work?

Now identify what things you really enjoy doing and the things you really don't like doing.

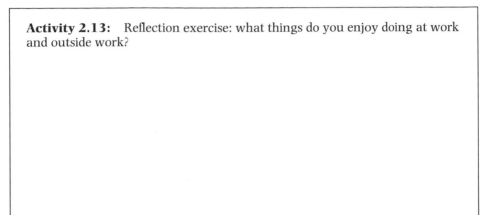

Activity 2.13: Reflection exercise: what things do you enjoy doing at work and outside work?

Activity 2.14: Reflection exercise: what things do you dislike doing at work and outside work?

Now you are ready to identify the 'Zone', your area of maximum performance. In it you work at your best because you are doing things that you both do well and also enjoy doing.

Activity 2.15:   Reflection exercise: what things do you enjoy doing *and* do well?

List here the things that you listed in both Activity 2.11 and 2.13.

Case study 2.1 continued

Angela Crossman finds that she really enjoys looking after people with chronic illnesses. As she gets to know them well she is able to do effective health promotion with them. She excels when she can relax with people because she has met them before, and she loves being able to teach them how to manage their illness better. She would like to do more teaching but that has not been possible as a practice nurse in her medical centre.

Where do you want to be?

There is no magical, perfect job waiting for you. There are a few jobs out there though that will give you a 'best fit'. These are jobs that suit you and stimulate and challenge you so that you perform naturally at your best. The effort is in finding and securing these jobs. What are you looking for? There are a lot of factors to put into the melting point. A lot of things need to be right for you before the job is right.

For example, the job must match your interests and move you closer to your bigger goals. If you need £35 000 a year to survive, that rules out quite a few jobs! If you have a time-consuming hobby, or children, hours of work will be important to you. Look at how the factors in Figure 2.2 overlap between the person themselves, their organisation and the job itself. Getting a best fit from all three perspectives should give you maximum stimulation, challenge and performance.

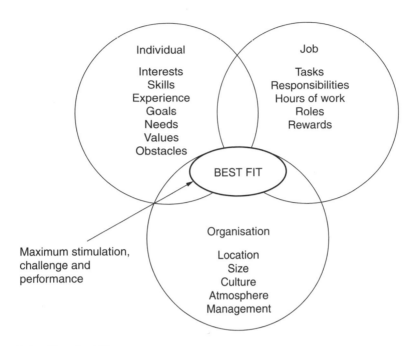

Figure 2.2: Your best fit.

What does your ideal working day look like?

If you could go to work tomorrow, not to your current job, but to a job created to be ideal for you, what would it consist of? Have a go at describing it. Do not worry about giving it a job title but describe the building blocks of the job that would make up your day.

Case study 2.1 continued

Angela would want an 8am start and a 3pm finish to her ideal working day as she has school age children. She would like to spend the morning running a chronic disease management clinic. She would like to have the opportunity of supervising a student attached to the practice and have time for a tutorial/ mentoring session every day. After an early lunch she would like to liaise with other practices on the best way to manage patients with specific chronic illnesses, then update her practice systems accordingly.

What kind of ideal day would you create for yourself? Complete Activity 2.16 (overleaf).

Activity 2.16: Reflection exercise: describe your ideal working day and its components

Your ideal working environment

The environment in which you work is as important as the job you do.

Case study 2.1 continued

Angela would ideally like to work in the country with less than 30 minutes to commute to work on traffic-free roads. She would like to work on her own but with other staff in the office, in a building with plenty of light and with a good delicatessen nearby! She would like to work with a high level of autonomy and very little supervision. Her ideal team should have altruistic ideals and not be driven by money and targets.

Now complete Activity 2.17.

Activity 2.17: Reflection exercise: where would you like to work ideally?

Location

Size of organisation

Continued

Values

Atmosphere

Nature or level of supervision

The next questions in Activities 2.18 and 2.19 are big ones and not easy to answer, but if you are not aware of what you really want you are probably not going to get your ideal job!

Activity 2.18:   Reflection exercise: what one thing do you want most from your career?

Now consider the following exercise.

Activity 2.19:   Reflection exercise: where do you want to be in:

3 months?

1 year?

5 years?

How are you going to get there?

Reaching your career goal may well involve changing jobs or taking a secondment, or assuming extended or additional roles in your current position. Identifying potential work opportunities can be difficult, but talking to colleagues can yield surprising results. You could also arrange to speak to someone with management responsibility or who works in another organisation who might be aware of suitable openings locally.

You might want to speak to someone who is currently working in the field in which you would like to develop. You can learn from their experience and find out more about their career development pathway. See if they are aware of any forthcoming opportunities or training in the field. Many NHS organisations have their own internal jobs market and regularly advertise vacancies – make sure you receive a copy of their vacancy circulars or look at their website every week.

Expand your horizons further by looking in local or national newspapers and professional journals to see what is available. If you are interested in a particular post but need to find out more before formally applying then make contact for more information – informal enquiries are often welcome. All this can take time and effort and can test your resolve about how serious you are about developing your career!

Give it a go for a few weeks then jot down all the opportunities you have come across in Activity 2.20.

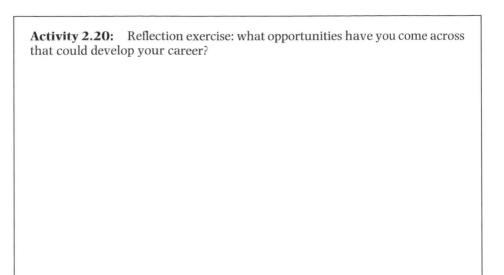

Activity 2.20: Reflection exercise: what opportunities have you come across that could develop your career?

Checking it out

For each possible opportunity that you have captured in Activity 2.20, do a more in-depth analysis in Activity 2.21, 2.22 or 2.23 of how that job would allow you to do the things that you are good at or suit your circumstances. We have allowed you three goes at this for three different opportunities. If you have written down more, photocopy Activity 2.23 as many more times as you need it. Circle the number that grades the various aspects of the potential job opportunity. This will help you to check out whether you are heading in the right direction with this particular career opportunity or not. It will also help you to identify what you need to do next.

Check out with people already doing similar jobs what skills they need to do the job well, what the job gives them, what the culture and management is like in that workplace. Is that what you are looking for?

Activity 2.21: Reflection exercise: career opportunity (first) you are considering

To what extent will this career opportunity:

	Not at all				*Significantly*
• allow you to do the things you are good at and enjoy?	1	2	3	4	5
• use your existing skills?	1	2	3	4	5
• develop new skills which you wish to acquire?	1	2	3	4	5
• give you what you want from work?	1	2	3	4	5
• motivate you?	1	2	3	4	5

- be suitable for you in terms of:
  - location?   1   2   3   4   5
  - size of organisation?   1   2   3   4   5
  - work culture?   1   2   3   4   5
  - supervision (nature, extent, of you/by you)? 1   2   3   4   5

What else do you need to find out about this career opportunity?

Activity 2.22:   Reflection exercise: career opportunity (second) you are considering

To what extent will this career opportunity:

	Not at all				*Significantly*
• allow you to do the things you are good at and enjoy?	1	2	3	4	5
• use your existing skills?	1	2	3	4	5
• develop new skills which you wish to acquire?	1	2	3	4	5
• give you what you want from work?	1	2	3	4	5
• motivate you?	1	2	3	4	5
• be suitable for you in terms of:					
– location?	1	2	3	4	5
– size of organisation?	1	2	3	4	5
– work culture?	1	2	3	4	5
– supervision (nature, extent, of you/by you)?	1	2	3	4	5

What else do you need to find out about this career opportunity?

Activity 2.23: Reflection exercise: career opportunity (third) you are considering

To what extent will this career opportunity:

	Not at all				*Significantly*
• allow you to do the things you are good at and enjoy?	1	2	3	4	5
• use your existing skills?	1	2	3	4	5
• develop new skills which you wish to acquire?	1	2	3	4	5
• give you what you want from work?	1	2	3	4	5
• motivate you?	1	2	3	4	5
• be suitable for you in terms of:					
– location?	1	2	3	4	5
– size of organisation?	1	2	3	4	5
– work culture?	1	2	3	4	5
– supervision (nature, extent, of you/by you)?	1	2	3	4	5

What else do you need to find out about this career opportunity?

Taking action

This is the hardest part. What stops you leaving a job that at best you find lacking in stimulation and at worst toxic in the way that it erodes you, leaving you feeling worn out, stressed and/or apathetic?

There are many reasons you stick by a job that logic tells you to leave. Often it is a lack of self-confidence. You doubt your ability to move to get a good job. You doubt your ability to transfer your skills. You repeat to yourself yearningly, 'what else could I do?'. You may not be fully aware of what your skills actually are. (So all the more reason to move on to Chapter 3 to undertake some more objective exercises to identify your skills and strengths.)

Another common reason for staying in a dissatisfying job is being too comfortable in your 'comfort zone'. Looking for a new job takes lots of your spare time and then the rest. Marketing and parading yourself around is embarrassing and exhausting. There are no guarantees that it will get you a job any better than the one you are already in.

Heavy financial commitments may hold you back if you are wanting to make a change in direction that involves less pay. Depression rears its head surprisingly often, purely because the wrong job can lead to depression, which will then rob you of the get up and go to find the right job for you.

Lack of support will stop you progressing. It is difficult to go through this process alone. Use your friends, family and colleagues if you can. Discuss career possibilities with them. Ask them to check out your responses to the reflection exercises in this chapter or involve them in further in-depth analysis in the next chapter. Have they got new insights about your strengths and weaknesses of which you were previously unaware?

Then there is that proverbial chestnut, fear of failure. What if it doesn't work out? What if you step from the familiar job to the less known and it goes wrong?

There will be obstacles in your pursuit of a fulfilling career. Of course there will. But you can refuse to let those potential barriers control your decisions. The main thing is to be aware which particular obstacle is yours. What are you up against here? What are you really afraid of? Are your fears rational? Are you maybe imagining a sequence like this: if you branch out into something new it will not work out, you will be unemployed and so you will not be able to pay the mortgage, so your partner will leave you? There are no guarantees in the pursuit of a job that really suits you, except that once successful you will look back and wish that you had made the move a lot earlier.

Remember that there is likely to be a constant conflict in you between the part of you that wants and drives change and the part of you that resists it (*see* Figure 2.3). There will be lots of things driving you to a goal such as interest and ambition. There will also be things stopping you from pursuing that goal. It's never too late to revise your career direction.

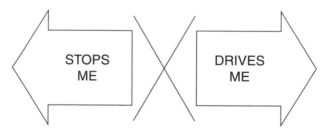

Figure 2.3:   Conflicting factors in your career direction.

It is worth teasing out what the drivers and resisters are for you that influence the speed or nature of a possible change in your career, as in Activity 2.24. This process can help you to reduce your resistance to change and strengthen your motivation to develop further.

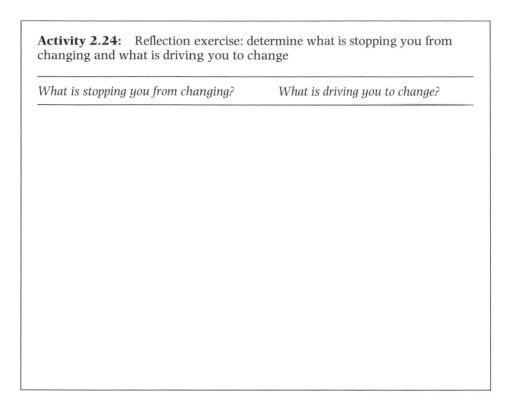

Activity 2.24:   Reflection exercise: determine what is stopping you from changing and what is driving you to change

What is stopping you from changing?   *What is driving you to change?*

Next steps

Once you have decided that you do indeed want to make a career change you need to plan how to do it. This is not as frightening as it seems.

Case study 2.1 continued

Angela does not need to rush and give up her job, but she does need to start finding out what possibilities exist for her. After talking to colleagues she thinks working as a nurse practitioner might suit her, either working for a primary care or hospital trust. She wants to find out more about what a clinical nurse specialist does and about nurses with specialist responsibility in hospital. Angela enjoys teaching so much that she wonders whether she should move into education, but is not sure where to start finding out about it. She needs to ask around to find out if anyone knows of any nurses who are doing a lot of teaching and speak to them. She can go to the local university and chat to one of the nurse lecturers there.

So she does not have to make any difficult decisions about her career yet but she does need to spend concentrated effort finding out about more about teaching opportunities and the qualifications needed.

How about you? You can make yourself a plan of action in Activity 2.25, such as ...

Activity 2.25: Reflection exercise: what practical steps do you need to take next?

	Practical step	By when?
1		
2		
3		
4		
5		

If you know where you want to go with your career and you are doing something active and practical about it, the decision will 'make itself' as you eliminate choices, come across new possibilities and clarify what it is you really want to do next. Then all you have to do is get on with it!

Do you have what it takes to get that job? If not, how do you get the skills and experience it takes? Finally, do you have the courage to stop thinking about how nice it would be if your job suited you better, used your skills better and was getting you where you wanted to go? Instead, do you have the courage to do something concrete about changing or developing your career?

3

Look in depth at your skills and strengths and where you are with your career

Ruth Chambers

So far much of the thinking you have done about what you want from an ideal or fulfilling career has come from you reflecting on what you think you do well or what you enjoy at work. Hopefully you did involve a colleague, friend or member of your family in checking out the series of reflection exercises in Chapter 2. But here is a further opportunity to try out some different approaches to analysing your career progress to date and think further about how you want to develop.

360° feedback[1]

This collects together perceptions from a number of different people who are relevant to your work, about you, as in Figure 3.1.

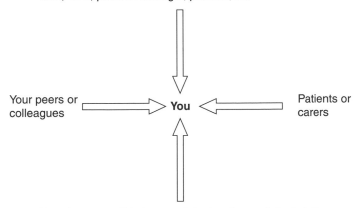

Figure 3.1: 360° feedback.

The wider the spread of people giving you feedback, the more rounded the picture. You could give a feedback questionnaire to at least three people in each of the groups above, who are all in a position to comment on your skills or strengths, or your potential areas for improvement. An independent person can then collect and collate the questionnaires and discuss the results with you. If you do this exercise as a team or group you have to take care that the learning experience is not spoilt by malicious comments against which individuals cannot readily defend themselves.

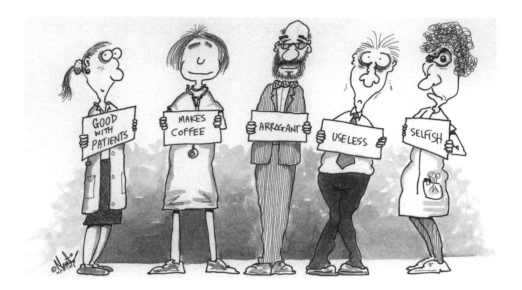

Self-assess or gain another person's perspective of your performance[1]

You might describe any aspect of your work as statements (A to G as in Activity 3.1) about your competence or performance as a self-assessment by marking the extent to which you agree on the linear scales opposite. For instance, if statement A was rewritten by you as: 'I am competent in a particular task (e.g. writing a protocol, implementing a strategy)', you could self-assess the extent to which you agree.

Alternatively, you could ask colleagues to fill in the assessment form about you. Objective feedback is usually more reliable than your own self-assessment, when you may have blind spots about your own performance. As you become more confident in this method of reviewing your competence, you might emphasise how consistent you are in your application of good practice – as in the statements opposite where we have sometimes included 'consistently', 'always' or 'usually'. You can set your own challenges.

If you have a mentor you might discuss and reflect on the completed marking grids with him or her.

Activity 3.1:   Marking grid: circle the number which represents your views or feelings about each statement – complete the grid on more than one occasion and compare results over time

A   I consistently treat colleagues politely and with consideration.

STRONGLY AGREE   to   STRONGLY DISAGREE

1----------------2----------------3----------------4----------------5----------------6

B   I am aware of how my personal beliefs could affect my management of the team, and take care not to impose my own beliefs and values.

STRONGLY AGREE   to   STRONGLY DISAGREE

1----------------2----------------3----------------4----------------5----------------6

C   I always treat colleagues and other staff equally and ensure that some groups are not favoured at the expense of others.

STRONGLY AGREE   to   STRONGLY DISAGREE

1----------------2----------------3----------------4----------------5----------------6

D   I try to maintain my relationship with the staff member when an issue has been resolved.

STRONGLY AGREE   to   STRONGLY DISAGREE

1----------------2----------------3----------------4----------------5----------------6

E   I always maintain confidentiality about other colleagues' personal business.

STRONGLY AGREE   to   STRONGLY DISAGREE

1----------------2----------------3----------------4----------------5----------------6

F   I usually involve colleagues and other staff in decisions relating to their work as far as possible.

STRONGLY AGREE   to   STRONGLY DISAGREE

1----------------2----------------3----------------4----------------5----------------6

Strengths, weaknesses (or challenges), opportunities and threats (SWOT) or (SCOT) analysis[2]

You can undertake a SWOT (or SCOT) analysis of your own performance, working it out on your own, or with a workmate or mentor, or with a group of colleagues. Brainstorm the strengths, weaknesses (or challenges), opportunities and threats of your role or circumstances.

Strengths and weaknesses (or challenges) of your roles might relate to your clinical knowledge or skills, experience, expertise, decision making, communication skills, interprofessional relationships, political skills, timekeeping, organisational, teaching or research skills. Opportunities might relate to your unexploited experience or potential strengths, expected changes in the NHS, or resources for which you might bid. For example, you might train for or set up a special interest post.

Activity 3.2:   Undertake a SWOT analysis of your career

Strengths   Weaknesses

Opportunities   Threats

Threats will include factors and circumstances that prevent you from achieving your aims for personal, professional or career development or service improvements. These might be to do with your health or time-limited investment by the primary care organisation (PCO) or trust.

List the important factors in your SWOT (or SCOT) analysis in order of priority. Draw up goals and a timed action plan for you to follow and involve colleagues as appropriate.

Draw up a force-field analysis[3]

This tool will help you to identify and focus down on the positive and negative forces in relation to your work. You will gain an overview of the weighting of these factors. Draw a horizontal or vertical line in the middle of a sheet of paper. Label one side 'positive' and the other side 'negative'. Draw bars to represent individual positive drivers that motivate you on one side of the line, and factors that are demotivating on the other negative side of the line. The thickness and length of the bars should represent the extent of the influence; that is, a short, narrow bar will indicate that the positive or negative factor has a minor influence and a long, wide bar a major effect. *See* Box 3.1 for an example.

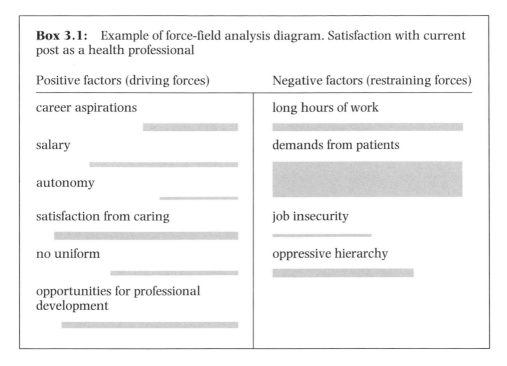

Box 3.1: Example of force-field analysis diagram. Satisfaction with current post as a health professional

Positive factors (driving forces) | Negative factors (restraining forces)

career aspirations | long hours of work

salary | demands from patients

autonomy |

satisfaction from caring | job insecurity

no uniform | oppressive hierarchy

opportunities for professional development

Take an overview of the resulting force-field diagram and consider if you are content with things as they are, or can think of ways to boost the positive side and minimise the negative factors. You can do this part of the exercise on your own, with a peer or in a small group in your workplace, or with a mentor or someone from outside your organisation. The exercise should help you to realise the extent to which a known influence in your life, or in the workplace as a whole, is a positive or negative factor. Make a personal or organisational action plan to create the situations and opportunities to boost the positive factors in your career and minimise the bars on the negative side.

Life line review[4]

Here is a reflective exercise that requires you to plot (on a timeline) the highs and lows of your career to date. It is amazing what you can learn about your relative strengths and weaknesses when you look back at how your career path has worked out. Why do you think you can diversify or develop your career now if you have not done that in the past? If your career has been in a rut at periods in your past, what can you do now to take up the career opportunities available and optimise developments for yourself? Adapt the dates on the timeline in Figure 3.2 for yourself. Then write some details of your career to date reflecting on the positives and negatives.

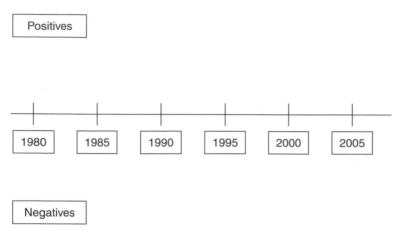

Figure 3.2:   Your timeline.

Questions to explore your timeline of experience

- Is there a pattern to the line?
- What do the turning points have in common?
- What sort of events were crises for you?

Take out a few instances and analyse each in depth. What were your circumstances at the time? What were the factors that restrained you from developing your skills or accelerating your career development then? What were the factors at the time that encouraged you or enabled you? You could look back at Box 3.1 and undertake a force-field analysis of each timeline experience.

Questions to pose to enable you to learn from the timeline experience and action plan

- What does the line tell you about your attitude to risk?
- Who are the people who have influenced your career to date?
- How have you managed change?
- What would you hope the line looks like when extended to 2008 or 2012 say?

Having reviewed your career to date consider what options exist for career development for you now. Make a plan that takes account of how you have behaved and coped with risk and change in the past.

Learndirect provides resources if you want to take stock and evaluate your skills from your early influences and decisions onwards.[5] Their workbook can facilitate you in identifying high and low points in your career.[5] It helps you to realise the skills and qualities you may be able to transfer from your experience, including your hobbies and leisure activities, to your career.

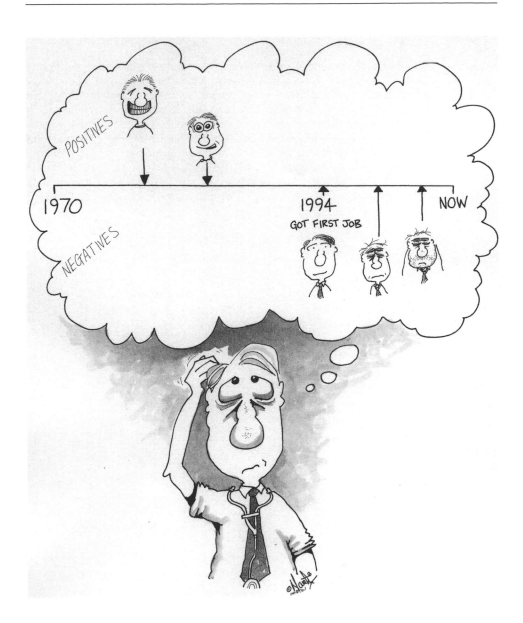

The GROW model[4]

The GROW (goal, reality, options, way forward) sequence is a simple way for you to consider change. This reflective exercise (Activity 3.3) will help you to be specific about your career goals. The emphasis on realism will help you to be clear about your options and what is possible for you. Then you can decide what you are going to do and when. You might do this exercise on your own or with a coach or mentor.

Considering career change is never easy and this approach starts with the positive; determining where you are trying to get to. Too often change starts with the problems and if you dwell on these barriers you may feel defeated before you have even started. If the change you are considering seems too big or complex you will need to begin with a small component of your goal, for example developing a particular skill or special interest.

Activity 3.3:   The GROW diagram for you to commit to a career plan of action

Step	Action (include timescales and milestones as appropriate)
Goal: Decide what you would you like to happen Decide what are your long-term aims	
Reality: Assess what is really happening at the moment Review any problems: with your job, your organisation or practice, your specialism or your profession, your work/life balance Work out what is missing in your career or your life Beware of any assumptions you are making	
Options: Cover the full range of career or life choices you have, and prioritise Brainstorm what different actions you could try to achieve your career goal	
Way forward: Plan which of these options you are going to do and how long it will take you and make a commitment Identify likely obstacles that might disrupt your plan and how to overcome them Seek support for your plan to increase the likelihood of it happening as you envisage	

Record any plans and changes in your personal development plan (PDP). Highlight your educational and development needs. Add timescales for your individual plan of action. Think how you will evaluate your progress and add those activities in too. Discuss your plan with your line manager at an individual performance review or with your appraiser. Revise your PDP and make further submissions for funding or career development accordingly.

What makes you think about leaving your current job[6]

If you're reviewing your career you may be thinking about leaving your current job, because you are dissatisfied with it, or because it is time for you to progress in your career. First reflect on whether you really do want to leave. You may be fed up with some other aspect of your life and be unfairly 'blaming' your job for the general unhappiness you feel. Here are a few prompts for you to probe what makes you think about leaving your job:

- what do you dislike about your current job?
- is it boredom, stress, work overload, relationships, the environment?
- how are these problems affecting you specifically?
- what would you like to do less of in your job?
- what would you like to do more of?
- have you been here before? Is the problem part of a pattern in your career?
- what will you be looking for in your next job or way of life if you leave?

There will be some good things about staying in your job too. There could be a great deal of disruption if you were to leave your current job; for instance, in relation to your regular income, job security, your work identity or status, familiarity with the organisation and its way of working, pensions, easy journey to and from work, workplace benefits such as childcare or nursery, your ability to do your job. So think about:

- what good things does your current job provide?
- what would you lose if you left?
- what frightens you about leaving your job?
- have you been here before? Is your reluctance to leave your current post a part of a pattern in your career?

Talk over your responses with a trusted mentor or friend or your partner at home and get their perspectives, allowing for their advice being biased by their own fears or reluctance to see you leave your current job.

Finding your balance[7]

Another way to think out more about what makes you tick or gives you a buzz is to complete the linear analogue scales overleaf. These are lines drawn between two opposite statements, which might describe your values, beliefs or preferences for the nature of your work. You could mark a cross where you feel you are for each. Or you might complete it now, store your markings away and compare with your responses in future, to understand how your career needs are changing over time. Or you might discuss your markings with someone else – a mentor or careers adviser perhaps.

Activity 3.4:   Defining your balance

Employment -- Occupation

Work -- Leisure

Status -- Interest

Creative --- Directed

Leading -- Supporting

Money -- Comfort

Solitude --- Team

Structure -- Fluidity

Near location --- Far location

Static -- Peripatetic

One organisation -- Portfolio

Find out more about your personality profile

You cannot make a rational choice about the type of career track you follow, without understanding the 'inner you' and what you have to offer. Your career and personality match are very important – and your personal preferences for your balance between work and leisure, work and income, degree of responsibility, type of work, and extent of interaction with people. Knowing more about yourself, your personality and emotions, will help you to interact with and manage other people better. Your feelings are highly influenced by your personality and your value system, all part of emotional intelligence.

Personality profile tests attempt to show individuals their preferred style of behaviour, in order that they can then choose the aspect of their profession that best matches the way they behave. Opinions about the benefits of psychometric testing are divided. The aim of the test is to identify a person's preferred way of behaving, based on their individual ways of perceiving the world and exercising judgement, in order to help in every aspect of life, career and personal relationships.

There are many varieties of personality profile questionnaires. Three of the best known are the Myers Briggs type indicator, the Sci45, and the 16PF questionnaire which assesses 16 personality factors. The Sci45 is a validated psychometric instrument designed by the Open University for selection of medical specialties by doctors in training. The Myers Briggs profile has four dimensions:

* E or I extroversion or introversion
* S or N sensing or intuition
* T or F thinking or feeling
* J or P judging or perceiving.

There is no right or wrong personality, just different personalities which work more or less effectively depending on the situation you are in. There is no ideal personality fit for a particular job, and a mix of different personalities within the same specialty or workforce group brings fresh perspectives and balances the work team. For many people, becoming more aware of their personal preferences and styles means that they gain confidence and pride in their own characteristics rather than seeking to conform to an imagined stereotype. Understanding yourself better helps you to find colleagues or teams where you are more likely to be compatible with the others, or the team character or workplace philosophy.

Some knowledge of your personality is necessary if you are to be helped to realise your potential. The shy, inward-looking person is not going to enjoy a work situation that calls for constant interaction, and the gregarious extrovert will become depressed if they are deprived of social contact. Understanding your own personal preferences and nature and what you want out of life should help you to develop an appropriate career path (*see* Box 3.2).

Box 3.2:   About personality type

- There is no right or wrong, better or worse combinations of personality types
- If you know more about your type you can understand yourself better
- Each person is unique
- Everyone uses each of their preferences to some degree
- The human personality is too complex for type to explain everything about you

---

Find out which facilitators or consultants can provide you with an analysis of your personality profile in your locality. Ask the education or learning lead in your trust for contact details or look for possibilities on the web. You may have to pay for a resource such as this yourself in a private capacity.

Self-analysis: your skills and strengths, plans and vision

Having worked through the reflection exercises in Chapter 2 and then the selection of in-depth exercises in this chapter you are now well placed to bring all the information together with this in-depth analysis. You might reflect on your career development and do this analysis by yourself, or work through it with a mentor, tutor or trusted colleague.

Who are you and where are you now?

Looking inwards

YOU
- What are your strengths and weaknesses in your various roles or posts?
- Do you understand your own personality: have you undertaken a personality profile test? Do the insights about your personality affect your career choice?
- What transferable skills do you have that might fit you for a different kind of career?

- How does your current work and life measure up to your inner values?
- What kind of roles and responsibilities do you prefer? Do you enjoy leading or following? Do you like to manage or be managed?
- What fears do you have that you need to overcome?
- What qualities do you have that you need to exploit or harness?

YOUR CURRENT JOB
- Do the features of your job fit with your personal style?
- How satisfied are you with your job – working hours, responsibility, location, patient contact, workload, income, challenge, opportunities for change or development, extent of socialising, your skills, on-call commitment, support from colleagues, variety?
- How satisfied are you with your career in general?
- What aspects of work do you value?
- Are there inner barriers that hinder your career advancement in your current job (e.g. self-doubt, low self-esteem)?
- Do you act the part in your post, even if you do not feel confident?
- Do you exceed your job description? You can impress others with your initiative and capability.
- Do you set yourself new targets within your job to keep your interest alive and provide new challenges?
- Do you nurture your relationships with other colleagues? You never know when you may need their support or help.

Looking outwards

- What opportunities are there for promotion or other roles or extending your skills, in your current job?
- What opportunities might there be for developing new skills or enhancing current skills in your present job?
- What other jobs are on offer elsewhere for which you might apply?
- What other role(s) and responsibilities do you see yourself taking on?
- Have you got enough support from others at work?
- What qualities and skills do others perceive that you have?
- Is your potential recognised or realised in your current post?

Looking sideways

- How do your current workload and conditions impact on your family and other aspects of your non-working life?
- How satisfied are you with your lifestyle and time spent outside work – sport, relaxation, hobbies, travel?
- How much quality time do you have for friends?
- What is the balance like between your current work and other aspects of your life?
- Do you have a mentor? A role model or influential colleague might well give your career a boost.

What changes do you want to make?

- To what extent are you content to remain in the same job, practice or NHS trust?
- To what extent will your current role satisfy you in one/three years' time – *see* Activities 3.5–3.7?
- What is it that you most want to achieve? What are your career goals?
- Do your career goals conflict with other types of success or fulfilment that you are seeking in other areas of your life (for instance, financial goals, social goals, leisure goals, personal goals in relation to your family)?
- What will be your strengths and skills and achievements by certain time milestones?
- How will you acquire those skills and experience in the meantime to develop your full potential? Skills developed outside work may be just as important as those developed as part of your job.
- What resources do you have to help you achieve your career goals?
- Consider applying for promotion to show others that you are motivated to progress your career.

Activity 3.5:   Take a career challenge in formulating your goals

What role do you see yourself doing in three, five, fifteen years' time? Think widely: academic career, research interest or audit, opportunities for teaching, location, preferences or hobbies, access to relatives, alternative and parallel clinical or management work, availability of cover by colleagues, supportive colleagues, sponsors and friends. Do you know of someone whose career pathway or roles you would like to emulate?

Activity 3.6:   Where do you want to be in ONE year's time? Write down your goals after reading through the career challenge in Activity 3.5

Looking inwards:

-
-
-

Looking outwards:

-
-
-

Looking sideways:

-
-
-

Activity 3.7:   Where do you want to be in THREE years' time? Write down your goals after reading through the career challenge in Activity 3.5

Looking inwards:

-
-
-

Looking outwards:

-
-
-

Looking sideways:

-
-
-

Activity 3.8:   How are you going to get there?

Work out the series of steps you will need to take over the next 12 months to achieve your one-year goals, and longer-term action for your three-year or even five- or fifteen-year goals. Think how to make things happen. To whom can you talk to get more information or advice? Who can you visit to see if their type of work appeals to you? Who can give you well-informed careers guidance or career counselling? How can you gain the preliminary achievements and experience that you need?

Getting ready to make a change
What do you need to do first?

- Further reflection and review of how satisfied you are with your career, your job, your life in general – as in the first three parts of this analysis.
- Discuss your satisfaction and options with others close to you – at home, your family and friends, work colleagues, trusted advisers and confidantes.
- Find out more information and facts about other careers or new skills.
- Ask someone for advice about opportunities in their field and what their jobs entail.
- Seek further careers information, careers advice or guidance.
- Make a list of your options and reflect (with someone whose opinion you value) on their relative advantages.

Are you ready to change?

- How positive are you about going ahead and making changes?
- Does what you are proposing fit with your ethics, values and boundaries?
- What is it that has limited you from making changes in the past? Have you overcome those constraints or barriers now?
- Are you clear about what interests and motivates you to work effectively?

So what will you do?

Make your plans happen with timetabled action
Think of:

* setting goals
* what new insights, knowledge, skills and attitudes you need to develop
* using your skills and experience
* your timetable
* how you will proceed
* support and resources you will need to make your plans come to fruition
* overcoming limiting factors – what risks you need to manage
* situations you may wish to influence – to prevent or provoke events or activities.

So what will you do?

Activity 3.9:   What will you do if you don't get what you want or hope for?

Write down your contingency plans, for instance:

* how could you change your current job so that you have more job satisfaction?
* re-evaluate your options. What is your 'second choice' alternative career path or career development?
* re-assess your previous goals and objectives
* what other skills might you develop within medicine or in your leisure time?
* could you get more balance into your life by building in more self-development time?
* think again if anyone else might help you through all your networks and contacts
* can you fit two different jobs into your life, working part-time on each?
* think again about what you really want out of life
* counter any self-defeating beliefs that you have uncovered in undertaking the review of your career
* adopt some better personal stress management in all sections of your life and work
* build up your support mechanisms – at work, with friends, with family and your partner at home.

So what could you do?

References

1 Chambers R, Tavabie A, Mohanna K and Wakley G (2004) *The Good Appraisal Toolkit.* Radcliffe Publishing, Oxford.

2 Chambers R, Wakley G, Iqbal Z and Field S (2002) *Prescription for Learning.* Radcliffe Medical Press, Oxford.

3 Chambers R, Mohanna K, Wakley G and Wall D (2004) *Demonstrating Your Competence 1. Healthcare teaching.* Radcliffe Medical Press, Oxford.

4 Garcarz W (2004) *Career Planning for GP Tutors.* 4 Health Limited, Birmingham.

5 Learndirect (2003) Discover your hidden talents. The Open University, Buckingham. www.learndirect-advice.co.uk

6 Houghton A (2004) Leaving your job: part 1. *BMJ Careers.* **6 March**: 93–4.

7 Peskett S and Empey D (2003) A career check for medical managers. *BMJ Careers.* **6 December**: s179–80.

4

Effective careers information, guidance and career counselling: how it can help you

Ruth Chambers

By now you should have a good idea about career planning in general and how it is relevant to you, and realise that learning and personal development are key. You will need to:

- be aware that you must continually develop yourself throughout your career
- take responsibility for managing your own learning and career development
- develop skills to learn from all your experiences.

You should have reflected on your skills and strengths and identified some weaknesses and obstacles that may impede the career path(s) you are planning to take. You will have found other people's perspectives of your achievements and strengths really useful when you have come to discuss the reflection exercises with them that were included in Chapters 2 and 3.

Once you know what you want to do there are many sources of careers information. If you still don't know what you want to do, you may need careers advice or guidance to direct you to the careers information and opportunities that are available. Or career counselling could help you to explore your strengths and discover different career and life options.

Careers information

Careers information gives you the facts about the qualifications and experience needed for alternative career pathways and the opportunities that there are for career progression. This includes written and/or verbal information about the number and type of posts available at various levels in particular specialties and fields, and details of the qualifications and training necessary.[1]

The national NHS Careers initiative in England provides much of the basic information about entry criteria and details of training for all type of careers in the health field. Paper and electronic information resources capture the individual experiences of health professionals describing their daily working lives. Or you could look at the website of NHS Professionals (*see* Box 4.1) for more ideas.

Box 4.1:   NHS Professionals www.nhsprofessionals.nhs.uk

NHS Professionals is a special health authority which is essentially a non-profit-making in-house staff agency for the NHS in England. It provides locum staff and keeps a register of their activity. The organisation manages temporary and flexible workers in the NHS, and supports these groups of staff, in an attempt to reduce their isolation.

The key to good career planning is information gathering from people, books, and general observation. By conducting your career by chance rather than thoughtful planning you end up taking opportunities as they happen along, rather than taking control and finding the best match of career for your own needs, preferences and experience.

There are some good books that describe the wide variety of jobs and opportunities available to health professionals, giving you ideas about what else you might try and how you might branch out – into a career in journalism, sports medicine etc.[1-3]

You should be able to get information about:

- the qualifications and opportunities about other similar posts or alternative specialties
- educational opportunities: bursaries, grants, new and established degree courses
- non-health careers (maybe being a clinician or manager in the NHS isn't so bad when you consider the other options?).

Careers advice or guidance

Careers advice or guidance is personal and directive and provides advice within the context of the opportunities that are available. It is useful for those who have not made a career decision or are unaware of the best way of achieving their career goals.

You might find it helpful to talk over where you are at with a careers adviser. This could be someone with a designated job in careers guidance. Or it could be a mentor, a friend or colleague, your old tutor or the local continuing professional development (CPD) tutor. Someone providing careers advice or guidance should know about, and be able to provide, advice within the context of the opportunities that are available to you as an individual.

Without adequate careers support you may remain ignorant of the options available, spend too much time in posts that are not ultimately relevant, and even be lost to the NHS altogether if you do not find the right niche for you.

The person giving you advice or guidance about your career should be well informed about options and opportunities for you, and their information or advice should not be biased. Line managers or equivalent for independent contractors may not give impartial advice to colleagues about their career development if they wish to retain staff in their current posts, or fill posts that fit with the trust's or practice's priorities. The quotes included in Box 4.2 show how line managers may have their own reasons for trying to retain staff in their current jobs, for instance.

Box 4.2: Examples of biased careers advice from line managers in one survey[1]

'I feel very strongly that people who have recently undertaken specialist training should have formal careers advice on a regular basis. This would help them to make better decisions about their future working lives. This may not come best from their line manager as they may have a vested interest in keeping people in their present situations.' (nurse)

'People (line managers etc) assume you want to remain in the profession you have chosen. They are not going to encourage you to change careers because of the risk of leaving your department short of staff. Many health professionals have been specifically trained for their job. I don't know what else I could do with a degree in occupational therapy without retraining (which has financial implications).' (occupational therapist)

Career counselling[4,5]

Career counselling is an intensive process requiring specialist skills. Career counselling is an umbrella term for the process of enabling somebody to evaluate their current situation and identify what steps are needed in order to change. It will usually include identification of a person's strengths and weaknesses in relation to their work options, and possibly bring in a variety of careers information.

The extent and type of help and support people need depends on their personal circumstances; career counselling may then be more appropriate than careers guidance. Career counselling has the potential to help health professionals and managers at all stages of their NHS careers, but may be particularly important for those thinking of returning to practice, people who are unhappy or dissatisfied with their careers, or staff who want to discuss flexible career paths rather than long-term commitments.

Career counselling is a process and not an event. It involves the career counsellor being alongside someone, listening to them carefully and supporting them as they work through their problems. This process should enable people to recognise and utilise their own resources to manage career-related problems and make career decisions.

In most respects career counselling is similar to any other kind of counselling in that it offers a framework for looking at problem situations and provides support to enable the person with the problem to undertake whatever changes they may decide to make. Successful career counselling will enable that person to identify the issues that need to be dealt with and mobilise the resources they need to improve matters. A well-trained career counsellor can help you to work out solutions to your difficulties as described in Box 4.3.

Box 4.3: Career counselling could help you to:

- think carefully about taking time out from your healthcare career
- re-evaluate your career choice and why you are considering a change
- re-assess whether you work part-time or full-time or retire early

---

> • match your strengths to a career specialty or way of working that suits you –
> e.g. taking on more responsibility, or extending your skills (e.g. becoming a
> practitioner with special interest or trying a secondment to management).

People need career counselling when:

* they are dissatisfied with their current job or career prospects
* they seem unable to solve their career dilemma by themselves, although they do
  usually have the resources to do so
* their thinking about their career is clouded, and they need to talk things through
  with someone who is independent and non-judgemental
* they are not responding to the usual motivators at work
* they seem unaware of the consequences of their poor performance or behaviour at
  work
* they are engaging in self-deprecating behaviour at work
* they are unaware of their talents and strengths at work.

Career counselling allows the person to tell their story, then to start thinking about
what would need to be in place for the situation to be improved, and finally to work out
an action plan to deliver those changes. Career counselling involves matching the
components of a job with a person's preferences, strengths and qualifications. The
match between the choice of career and personality are very important and dictate
personal preferences for the balances between work and leisure, work and income,
degree of responsibility, type of work and extent of interaction with people. People
come for career counselling because they seek change, and most people have the
utmost difficulty changing aspects of their thinking and their lives.

The stages of career counselling are getting people to think through the following
sequence of challenges:

* 'Who am I and where am I now?'
* 'How satisfied am I with my career and my life?'
* 'What changes would I like to make?'
* 'How do I make them happen?'
* 'What do I do if I don't get what I want?'

Any successful action plan needs a timescale and a description of what is possible in
the short, medium and long term. The outcome of career counselling should be action.

Find a well informed careers adviser or career counsellor

Careers advisers and career counsellors should be well informed and skilled and offer
impartial help. It is increasingly being realised that careers advice and counselling
services should be available and accessible to all staff in the NHS at all stages of their
careers. You will want a careers adviser with a wide-based knowledge of what external
resources exist to which you may be referred for more detailed help or advice about
particular jobs or training opportunities.

Sometimes the same person is expected to be a mentor, educational supervisor, line
manager and careers adviser or counsellor to one individual, and conflicts of interest

can arise. If someone acting as your careers adviser or counsellor has line management authority over you, you are unlikely to trust in their independence. Worse still, they may act on their acquired insider knowledge of you on a future occasion if for example they are undertaking an appraisal with you or giving you a reference.

Activity 4.1:   Reflection exercise: do you know where you could obtain careers advice or guidance or career counselling?

Think back – have you ever received such help? yes/no

If so was it from someone who was experienced, who was well informed and gave you impartial advice, and who had dedicated time to spend with you?

Do you know where to get such careers information, advice or counselling from? Does your trust employ careers advisers or counsellors? Does your local further education college have a generic careers adviser whom you might see, or might they advise you where other professional career advice is available?

Find a mentor, coach or buddy

You will be more likely to follow your career action plans and overcome hiccups in the progress of your career if you have a trusted friend or adviser with whom to discuss your career path.

Seek a mentor[6]

A mentor relationship is more of a one-way relationship where the mentor has the time and capacity to listen to you and help facilitate you in making decisions about your career. Some mentors are only concerned with helping the person being mentored (the mentee) to identify and meet their educational or training needs through a development plan, whereas others give practical or emotional support too.

The emphasis is on the mentor helping the mentee to develop their own thinking and find their own way, not to teach the mentee new skills or act as a patron to ease the mentee's career path by special favours.

A mentor helps the person being mentored to realise their potential by acting as a trusted senior counsellor and experienced guide on personal, professional and educational matters. A mentor should be able to agree learning objectives with a mentee and subsequently guide the mentee to address their educational needs, identify their strengths and weaknesses, explore options with them, act as a challenger, encourage reflection and provide motivation. Your relationship with your mentor should be one of mutual trust and respect in a supportive yet challenging relationship where they remain non-judgemental.

You will start by agreeing ground rules for meeting – confidentiality, commitment, duration and frequency of sessions, location, the purpose, personal boundaries and how or whether you will record your meeting. Clarify the objectives and outcomes that you both want to cover. A common framework used for mentoring follows three stages:

1 *exploration*: when the mentor listens, prompts the mentee with questions
2 *new understanding*: when the mentor listens and challenges the mentee, recognises the strengths and weaknesses of the ideas, shares experiences, establishes priorities, identifies development needs, gives information and supportive feedback
3 *action planning*: encourages new ways of thinking, helps the mentee reach a solution, agree goals and decide action plans.

A mentor and mentee may be from different backgrounds and the differences may provoke a cross-fertilisation of ideas and shared understanding and perspectives. The mentoring session may be an opportunity to reinforce or analyse what learning took place after actually doing a new task or activity such as a secondment.

A coach could be what you need[6,7]

A coach could offer more directive help about your career in the same way that a sports coach urges an athlete on. Coaches work through one-to-one conversations in person or by email or telephone.

A good coach will be a successful motivator, be very supportive, establish a good rapport with the person being coached, be able to give constructive feedback and set clear objectives. The coach may be the learner's manager or tutor, unless an external coach is being employed. The coach will stretch and challenge you and encourage you to solve problems and make changes by yourself. A good coach is analytical rather than critical and is able to depersonalise the problems discussed in coaching sessions by focusing on facts, outcomes and performance rather than your personality or style.

Coaching involves a combination of psychology, business and communication skills. It consists of a partnership between coach and 'client' to clarify the client's goals for work and life and plan how to achieve those goals. The interactive relationship enhances your potential and performance to a greater extent than seemed possible when functioning on your own. Coaching is sometimes confined to learning a specific skill for a future event such as a job interview or presentation at a conference. At other times coaching might be more centred on the person as a whole, to help them progress more quickly with their professional and career development. Every coaching situation is different as each coach has their own particular style of working, and each client has their individual circumstances and is at a particular point in their life.

A professional or 'executive' coach generally has a minimum of five years' experience as a coach and a professional qualification such as in clinical psychology or occupational psychology, a diploma in counselling, Master Practitioner in Neuro Linguistic Programming or psychotherapy. Such an experienced coach will have expert knowledge of leadership and management behaviour, know about theory and practice of organisational behaviour and human psychology, be accredited to use personality profile testing and other personal assessment techniques, and have many interpersonal skills.

Coaching usually starts with an evaluation of your current effectiveness and your use of time and your priorities. Your coach will encourage you to reflect on how you might build on your strengths to change your current situation. They will enable you to overcome often self-imposed limitations that are stopping you from progressing as far or as fast as you might otherwise do. Your developing self-awareness and insight gradually built up should lead to lasting change.

> If you want to climb mountains and not level off, think bigger and take risks. (good advice from an established coach)

Outcomes of coaching vary depending on the circumstances of the person being coached. He or she may tackle their job more effectively and enthusiastically having clearer objectives. They may reorganise or change their situation at work so that they perform better, or re-evaluate their career and decide to find a different job.

> During the coaching, people gradually connect with their true ambitions and identify what steps are needed to achieve them. They gain more control of their lives and feel less tossed about by events. The feedback we get later from clients confirms that this is truly the case.[7]

A typical framework for a coaching session might be to:

- hear what's happened since last meeting
- agree the topics to work on
- agree what should be achieved by the end of the session
- agree priorities if there are too many issues
- undertake problem solving for each priority issue
- discuss what is the issue and why it is important
- discuss what has been tried already
- agree what would be an ideal state
- debate what's preventing the ideal state from happening now
- establish the extent to which you are preventing the ideal state from being achieved
- explore the options for resolving your problems
- discuss what skills are needed for your preferred option
- agree your strategy and target(s)
- select appropriate training methods
- make a realistic timetable for the training you have both agreed.

Find your buddy[6]

A buddy is someone in a similar situation to you with whom you have a reciprocal relationship, who gives you unconditional peer support. If your relationship with your buddy is successful you may keep in touch all your working lives.

You and your buddy might meet regularly for you to listen to each other, give practical or emotional support, swap information and identify possible solutions.

Although the relationship may be informal, you should formalise arrangements to meet, or your discussions will become snatched friendly chats rather than meaningful exchanges. You should each take turns at actively listening to the other, challenging when appropriate, giving constructive and supportive feedback as necessary.

You and your buddy should feel that you are on equal terms and have a mutual regard for each other's opinion. You should trust the other to preserve confidentiality about the issues you discuss.

References

1 Chambers R, Mohanna K and Field S (2000) *Opportunities and Options in Medical Careers.* Radcliffe Medical Press, Oxford.

2 Krechowiecka I (2002) *The A–Z of Careers and Jobs* (10e). The Times, Kogan Page, London.

3 Ward C and Eccles S (2001) *So You Want to be a Brain Surgeon?* (2e). Oxford University Press, Oxford.

4 Rogers C (1999) *Client Centred Therapy.* Constable, London.

5 Egan G (1990) *The Skilled Helper* (6e). Brooks Cole Publishing Co, New York.

6 Mohanna K, Wall D and Chambers R (2004) *Teaching Made Easy* (2e). Radcliffe Medical Press, Oxford.

7 Parsloe E and Wray M (2003) *Coaching and Mentoring.* Kogan Page, London.

5

Developing the workforce through the 'skills escalator' and Agenda for Change

Anne Longbottom

In this chapter we are going to look at how careers can be developed in the NHS and the initiatives that are being put in place to ensure that everyone who works with and for the NHS has the opportunity to develop their strengths and address their areas of weakness. So how can this tall order be achieved?

The skills escalator

The NHS Plan set out a vision for a modern health service designed around the patient's journey.[1] It focused on how redesigning services, employing more staff and introducing different working practices can improve the patient's experience. The 'skills escalator' strategy was set out to provide a vision for a new way of encouraging those in the workforce to develop and extend their careers.[2,3] This strategy describes the underpinning high-quality learning and development opportunities that are needed to realise the *NHS Plan*. It is key to supporting the development of a growing and changing workforce.

It is an exciting time if you are already working for or wish to join the NHS. Staff are being encouraged to constantly review and renew their skills and knowledge through lifelong learning. The skills escalator is about helping you to develop to be the best you can within your trust or practice, as part of a fulfilling career. You may wish to extend your skills at your current level of responsibility or choose to develop the skills necessary for the next level of responsibility or skill set. There is no guarantee of promotion or advancement from your current post even when you have gained the requisite knowledge and skills. But you should then able to take advantage of openings as they appear elsewhere.

Activity 5.1:   Reflection exercise: consider the job role that you would like to achieve

- What experience or qualifications do you need to undertake the role you would like to gain?
- How can you find out more about that particular role?
- What learning might you need to undertake to fulfil your career ambitions?

How does the skills escalator work?

There are seven levels in the skills escalator starting with people coming into work for the first time, rising to the most senior management roles such as chief executives or senior clinicians such as hospital consultants. How quickly you move up the skills escalator depends on your personal strengths and needs and those of the organisation: your trust, department or practice. These will change over time. Your age, background and existing academic attainments should no longer be a barrier to your career progress, if you have the drive and potential to progress in your career.

There will still be traditional entry points such as those for registered health professionals such as doctors, nurses, allied health professionals and others. But these will be complemented by other entry routes such as cadet schemes and role conversion, attracting people into the NHS from non-health careers who are seeking new challenges, and drawing qualified and experienced people back into the NHS workforce. The skills escalator concept does not mean that anybody can start as a porter and end up as a medical consultant but rather that you as an individual working for the NHS have the opportunity to develop through learning. Sometimes you will be stepping off and on the skills escalator as your personal situation dictates, but be constantly developing at a pace that fits your needs and ability.

What is Agenda for Change?[4]

Agenda for Change is the new pay and grading system for the NHS and replaces existing pay and conditions structures. It is the largest change to NHS pay and conditions since the health service was formed in 1948 and Agenda for Change was rolled out across the NHS from December 2004. The agreement applies to all staff directly employed by NHS trusts across the UK (including health and personal social services organisations in Northern Ireland), except very senior managers and staff within the remit of the Doctors' and Dentists' Review Body. So independent contractors in primary care such as dentists, optometrists, GPs and pharmacists and the staff they employ are not covered by Agenda for Change. It will allow the whole of the workforce employed by NHS trusts (with some exceptions) to be on the same pay band if they are doing different jobs which are of the same value.

There are three pay spines for:

1   staff covered by the Doctors' and Dentists' Review Body
2   staff covered by the extended remit of the Pay Review Body for Nursing and Other Health Professionals
3   other directly employed NHS staff with the exception of the most senior managers.

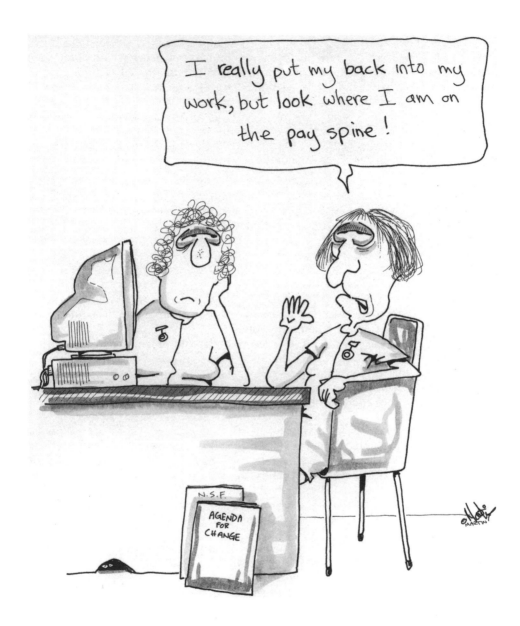

The agreement introduces new, single pay spines for the second and third of these groups, replacing the large number of separate occupational pay spines currently in existence. The second and third pay spines are divided into nine pay bands and all staff covered by this agreement were, on assimilation (the process by which staff are transferred from their existing pay structure to the new Agenda for Change pay structure), assigned to one of the pay bands on the basis of job weight as measured by the NHS Job Evaluation Scheme. Hundreds of jobs were evaluated and national job profiles drawn up, and the job evaluation score agreed. If a job matched one of these profiles it was assimilated on the basis of the profile score. If not, the job was analysed and evaluated locally at a review to produce a locally agreed job profile.

There are several pay points within each pay band. As you develop your knowledge and skills you will normally progress through one pay point each year up to the maximum in your pay band. At two defined 'gateways' in each pay band, you will only progress through the 'gateways' if you can demonstrate you have the knowledge and skills required. Staff who work in posts where recruitment and retention is difficult will be able to receive an additional premium as part of their pay.

The *Job Evaluation Handbook* sets out the basis of job evaluation.[5] The factors upon which jobs have been evaluated include:

- *communication and relationship skills*: where the highest level concerns 'providing and receiving highly complex, sensitive or contentious information where there are significant barriers to acceptance which need to be overcome using the highest level of interpersonal and communication skills'
- *knowledge, training and experience*: where the highest level involves 'advanced theoretical and practical knowledge of a range of work procedures and practices' or 'specialist knowledge over more than one discipline/function acquired over a significant period'
- *analytical and judgemental skills*: where the highest level consists of 'judgements involving highly complex facts or situations, which require the analysis, interpretation and comparison of a range of options'
- *planning and organisational skills*: where the highest level concerns 'formulating long-term, strategic plans which involve uncertainty and which may impact across the whole organisation'
- *physical skills*: where the highest level requires 'physical skills where a high degree of precision or speed and the highest levels of hand, eye and sensory co-ordination are essential'
- *responsibilities for patient/client care*: where the highest level is 'corporate responsibility for the provision of a clinical, clinical technical or social care service(s)'
- *responsibilities for policy and service development implementation*: where the highest level demands 'corporate responsibility for major policy implementation and policy or service development, which impacts across or beyond the organisation'
- *responsibilities for financial and physical resources*: where the highest level is of 'corporate responsibility for the financial resources and physical assets of an organisation'
- *responsibilities for human resources*: where the highest level involves 'corporate responsibility for the human resources or HR function.
- *responsibilities for information resources*
- *responsibilities for research and development*
- *freedom to act*: where the highest level involves the interpretation of 'overall health service policy and strategy, in order to establish goals and standards'
- *physical effort*
- *mental effort*: where the highest level requires 'intense concentration'
- *emotional effort*: rating frequency and intensity of exposure to distressing or traumatic circumstances
- *working conditions*: rating exposure to unpleasant working conditions or hazards.

Describing and rating jobs using these factors enables a much clearer definition of the roles and responsibilities of a post, as job titles may be misleading. There are many jobs where the job description is unique and has evolved to a fill a local service need.

Job evaluation

Job evaluation profiles and job descriptions are two different things and should not be confused. Job evaluation is:

- a system for comparing different jobs
- the basis for grading jobs in the new pay structure
- logical, consistent and systematic
- transparent.

It measures jobs and not people and is based on the demands of a particular job.
It is not:

- an assessment of people's skills – that is the remit of the Knowledge and Skills Framework
- an assessment of your performance
- a workload measurement tool.

You should have an up-to-date, agreed job description.[6] Not only is this good human resources practice, it also ensures that both you and your line manager have a common understanding of what is required in your job. A job description is generally set out in the form of a list of job duties.

Activity 5.2:   Update and agree your job description with your line manager

Do you have an up-to-date job description?

If not, you should sit down and think about what duties you currently undertake and compare this to your original job description.

If you find this difficult you could keep a diary for two or three weeks to see which duties and tasks you regularly perform and then arrange to discuss this with your line manager to agree revisions to your job description.

You could also discuss your job description with other people who have similar job roles and see how theirs compares with yours.

In addition to a job description it is also good practice to have a person specification. This is a list of qualities that an ideal candidate would possess if applying for the job, your post in this case. Some qualities might be desirable while others are essential. For example if you were to be employed in an administrative or clerical role it is essential that you can use a computer and type letters, but it might only be desirable for you to use a full range of software packages such as PowerPoint, Access or Excel.

> **Activity 5.3:**   Review the job specification describing your post with your line manager
>
> Does your job description have a person specification attached to it?
>
> If not, what qualities would you expect a person doing your job to have?
>
> If you do have a person specification, does it need updating in the light of the skills and experience someone in your current post would need?

There is no standard format for a job description. The format and content are for each individual trust or practice to agree as being appropriate to the needs of the organisation.

The NHS Knowledge and Skills Framework (KSF)

In order to assess what knowledge and skills you will need to undertake a specific role effectively, the NHS Knowledge and Skills Framework (KSF)[7] has been developed.
   'The purpose of the KSF is to:

*   facilitate the development of services so that they better meet the needs of users and the public through investing in the development of all members of staff
*   support the effective learning and development of individuals and teams – with all members of staff being supported to learn throughout their careers and develop in a variety of ways, and being given the resources to do so
*   support the development of individuals in the post in which they are employed so that they can be effective at work – with managers and staff being clear about what is required within a post and managers enabling staff to develop within their post
*   promote equality for and diversity of all staff – with every member of staff using the framework, having the same opportunities for learning and development open to them and having the same structured approach to learning, development and review.'[7]

This framework consists of six core dimensions, which you will do in your job at a level between 1 to 4. Level 1 describes dealing on a one-to-one basis in the relevant dimension (e.g. you and a patient), rising steadily to level 4, which relates to dealing with very complex matters and is likely to include corporate responsibility. There are 24 other specific dimensions, some of which you will do at varying levels depending on the nature of your role and responsibilities. These are listed on page 73, shown there as being integrated within your personal development plan (PDP).
   The KSF profiles of a job will act as a prompt for action by you and your manager at your annual appraisal, to ensure that your knowledge and skills about your current job are up to date. You will review your opportunity for personal and professional development. This may be to complement the work you currently undertake or prepare you for another role to help you progress in your career that will benefit the service. It will also enable you to see what knowledge and skills are required for future career steps, and identify the development you will need to support your progress on your career path.

The KSF is the NHS commitment to you as a member of staff to your learning and development. There also needs to be a commitment from you as an employee to ensure that you use these opportunities to benefit your practice or department and the people who use your services. These are shown in a variety of ways for example through personal commitment to your job, positive attitudes to work, professional behaviour when dealing with service users and other members of staff.

Activity 5.4:   Work out how the KSF is matched to the requirements of your role

Take a copy of the outline for KSF from the web address.[7] Which dimensions do you think apply to your job role other than the six core dimensions?

Now look at the Levels 1–4 for each of the six core and the other dimensions you have specified for your job. Which level do you think applies to each of those relevant to your job role?

You might be working at one level for one dimension and another level in a different dimension. This is quite acceptable and indicates the diversity of your role.

Finally, think of the positive attributes that you have which will assist in developing your role.

In order to progress through the pay band you must prove that you have continued to develop your knowledge and skills and kept up to date with current thinking in your field.

You will show the evidence for this learning and how you have applied it, through annual development reviews to produce a PDP. The review will take place between yourself and your line manager (or continuing professional development (CPD) tutor in some local areas) and should build on existing practice related to your current role, as well as looking at your professional and personal development in specific ways:

- how the duties and responsibilities of your job are being undertaken based on current agreed objectives
- application of your knowledge and skills in your workplace
- your consequent personal development needs taking into account your short- and long-term career development needs.

Use your PDP to anticipate what knowledge and skills you will need to progress through the gateways in your pay band.

What is a personal development review (PDR)?

A PDR is a process that links individual professional and personal development with the development of the organisation you work for. A PDR may be enveloped within your annual appraisal with your line manager or other person, or be held as a separate event.

Your employer has a responsibility to ensure that all staff in your organisation:

- understand their roles and what is expected from them
- are set appropriate, realistic, achievable targets (in consultation with individual members of staff)
- are given feedback as to how they are performing in their jobs, and an opportunity to reflect and comment on their own performance and that of their employing organisation
- are given appropriate training and development to help them become more effective in their jobs.

The central point of your PDR is a meeting with your line manager. This meeting will give your manager an opportunity to acknowledge the success and progress you have made, discuss any areas of concern or where there might be room for improvement, and confirm that your job description and KSF outline are up to date. Independent contractors without a line manager may make other arrangements with appraisers or CPD tutors.

You should be able to feed back any issues or concerns on the way you are managed or deployed and the organisation as a whole. The conversation should give you the opportunity to share ideas and discuss your own performance. Both the reviewer and reviewee should be well prepared for the review meeting to make it meaningful and effective.

Content of your personal development plan

Your trust or other professional body will no doubt have a recommended template that you can use to prepare and update your PDP ready for your appraisal. Some of the key sections that it should include comprise:

- your job description, matched against the core and specific dimensions of the KSF as relevant to your post, with the expected levels. You may have compiling or updating this as a job to do at your personal development review
- record and review of where you are up to with statutory and mandatory training compared with those deemed essential or desirable for your role
- a copy of your PDP from the previous year and how you have addressed the learning and development needs you prioritised last year. You could divide the evidence of your learning and how it has been applied under core headings such as: management, professional requirement, national or local policy, personal development, organisational priority – depending on the nature of your job
- an outline of priorities for your PDP for the coming year. Identify your learning needs through self-completion checklists, discussion, appraisal, audit, patient feedback. Are these personal or professional priorities, ones stemming from your trust or practice, local priorities or local or national policy?
- collecting any baseline information about your performance that you can use to justify why the topics you highlight are a priority and show your knowledge and skill gaps, or to use to demonstrate improvements after you have undertaken your planned learning and development activities and gathered information about similar aspects of your performance at a future date
- draft of your personal development plan ready to discuss at your appraisal, with learning objectives, expected outcomes, a range of types of learning activities, nature of resources you need and how you will obtain them, and the projected

timescale. Mention who will be included in your PDP (anyone other than you – doctors, members of your team, patients?). Think how you might integrate the core and specific dimensions of the KSF that are relevant to your post, into your PDP. You might define your learning needs and priorities for personal development against individual dimensions listed in Box 5.1

Box 5.1: Core and specific dimensions of the NHS Knowledge and Skills Framework (KSF)

Core Dimension 1	Communication
Core Dimension 2	Personal and people development
Core Dimension 3	Health, safety and security
Core Dimension 4	Service improvement
Core Dimension 5	Quality
Core Dimension 6	Equality and diversity
Dimension HWB 1	Promotion of health and wellbeing and prevention of adverse effects on health and wellbeing
Dimension HWB 2	Assessment and care planning to meet health and wellbeing needs
Dimension HWB 3	Protection of health and wellbeing
Dimension HWB 4	Enablement to address health and wellbeing needs
Dimension HWB 5	Provision of care to meet health and wellbeing needs
Dimension HWB 6	Assessment and treatment planning
Dimension HWB 7	Interventions and treatments
Dimension HWB 8	Biomedical investigation and intervention
Dimension HWB 9	Equipment and devices to meet health and wellbeing needs
Dimension HWB 10	Products to meet health and wellbeing needs
Dimension EF 1	Systems, vehicles and equipment
Dimension EF 2	Environments and buildings
Dimension EF 3	Transport and logistics
Dimension IK 1	Information processing
Dimension IK 2	Information collection and analysis
Dimension IK 3	Knowledge and information resources
Dimension G 1	Learning and development
Dimension G 2	Development and innovation
Dimension G 3	Procurement and commissioning
Dimension G 4	Financial management
Dimension G 5	Services and project management
Dimension G 6	People management
Dimension G 7	Capacity and capability
Dimension G 8	Public relations and marketing

- consider how you might work towards your career aspirations or hopes for a more senior or different post that you want to achieve – within your PDP:
    - investigate through research in journals, books, on the internet the qualifications for other jobs that you find interesting

- ask the HR department for job descriptions and KSF profiles of the posts that interest you to see what are the essential and desirable skills required, and what the role entails
- speak to people within the department or area of work that you find interesting to find out about the day-to-day job role
- look for a secondment or opportunities to deputise for a manager
- be prepared to put yourself out to gain the opportunities to progress

   there will be lots more ways that you can think of, but remember that although the KSF will give you the opportunities for learning and development, you need those extra personal qualities and commitment to make things happen in your career. Anticipate barriers to what you intend to learn and plan how to overcome them
- evaluate what you have learnt and the extent to which you have applied your learning in practice or it has taken you along your career path
- note down how you will disseminate the learning from your plan to the rest of your team and patients, as appropriate. Reflect on whether you shared the outputs of last year's PDP with others or could still do so.

Once you have thought about the above prompts and questions you will have a good basis on which to plan and achieve your future learning and career goals and make the most of opportunities to progress within your chosen career.

References

1 Department of Health (2000) *The NHS Plan: a plan for investment, a plan for reform.* Department of Health, London. www.dh.gov.uk/publicationsandstatistics

2 Department of Health (2004) *Skills Escalator Resource Pack: achieving your potential.* Department of Health, London. www.dh.gov.uk/publicationsandstatistics

3 Department of Health (2001) *Working Together, Learning Together – a framework for lifelong learning for the NHS.* Department of Health, London. www.dh.gov.uk

4 Department of Health (2004) *Agenda for Change – what will it mean for you?* Department of Health, London. www.dh.gov.uk

5 Department of Health (2004) *Job Evaluation Handbook* (2e). Department of Health, London. www.dh.gov.uk

6 Department of Health (2004) *NHS Shadow Staff Council Job Description and Agenda for Change FAQs.* Department for Health, London. www.dh.gov.uk

7 Department of Health (2004) *The NHS Knowledge and Skills Framework and Development Review Guidance – Working Draft* Version 7. Department of Health, London. www.dh.gov.uk

6

Flexible working and portfolio careers

Ruth Chambers

Flexible working

Flexible working may be a good way of counteracting burnout. It may help you to keep your creativity and enjoyment of NHS work alive if working day after day in a frontline health setting is debilitating for you. You may just want to earn extra money by taking on additional work outside your core job, or keep your options open with a variety of jobs until you focus down on a particular area at some time in the future.

Activity 6.1: Reflection exercise: decide whether increasing the flexibility of your current post might suit you

How flexible is your working day or working week? Would you prefer that it was more flexible than it is?

If so, what could you do to adapt your working hours or work pattern to allow you to accommodate other work activities (tick all that apply):

- reduce hours and seek additional job outside the practice or trust
- change hours to liberate more blocks of time for other work (e.g. switch to starting earlier, ending later)
- find a job-sharer for your current post
- change jobs to one with more flexibility
- find work that can be done in your spare time from home (e.g. writing, own business)?

Many of those working in minimally part-time posts feel isolated within their work-places, especially if their working hours mean that coffee breaks and staff meetings do not coincide with times when other colleagues are free. Protected study time for group education with peers or the rest of the team can guard against such isolation.

It's all about choice – agreeing working hours that suit your income needs, with enough time off to spend with your partner and kids at home or for leisure. You will need sufficient spare time to recover from a difficult job, especially if you have a disability. Flexible working patterns require flexibility from your employer and colleagues as much as you yourself. The success of any innovative working arrangement depends as much on the willingness and positive attitudes of everyone involved to make the new arrangements work, as on the structure put in place to accommodate that work. One drawback to flexible working that is rarely realised until after the change has been made is the detrimental effect that the person's lesser availability in the workplace has on continuity. If you are a frontline clinician, patients can protest quite vociferously about your lack of availability, making you feel guilty and regret the loss of 'continuity of care' you had all previously taken for granted. If you are a manager, staff may feel rudderless at times you are not there and you will have to delegate and set up good cover arrangements.

Box 6.1:   Flexible working schemes

For information contact NHS Professionals on +44 (0)845 60 60 345.

Try a portfolio career

The possibility of combining one or more job roles or even two or more jobs held in parallel has often cropped up in the earlier chapters of the book. A portfolio career describes how you might mix and match various posts. The portfolio description implies that the skills involved in the mix of jobs are transferable. It may be that you combine a number of clinical specialties or add in management, law, education, the media etc. Use the reflection exercise in Activity 6.2 to think more deeply about why you want to develop a portfolio career rather than stick single-mindedly with an unchanging career path.

Activity 6.2:   Reflection exercise: consider what you would like to change about the features of your current job by converting to a portfolio career

This review exercise will help you to balance the mix of jobs you include in your future portfolio and what kind of mix of posts could make the change worthwhile. Consider:

- what it is that motivates you with your work – are there three key things?
- how satisfied you are with the amount of money you earn – do you want or need to earn more, taking your current outgoings into account?
- how content you are with the balance between your level of income and free time – how do you want to change the present balance?
- how often you use the range of your skills, knowledge and experience. Which of these do you want to develop or use more than in your present situation?
- how often you meet up with, or network with, like-minded colleagues – do you want to increase this side of your life?

Anyone of any age and at any stage in their career may consider embarking on a portfolio career. You might be starting out in a regular post with other powerful interests that you want to develop – academic or competing in a sport, maybe. You might be a dissatisfied clinician in mid-career and be seeking variety and more expertise. You might be in your 50s and thinking of diversifying before retirement.

The strengths of a portfolio career are the flexibility, variety, personal development and ability to react to new opportunities or changing circumstances – either your personal ones or in relation to your practice or your NHS organisation. It is far better to seize the opportunities while you are on top of your job and starting to need variety and new challenges rather than wait until you are starting to burn out from a constant overload of work.

First steps: taking stock before you change to a portfolio career

This may be your first opportunity to take stock of your career and try something different. You could include reasonably secure and well paid posts in your portfolio, or take a risk. For example, as well as part-time general practice, you could retrain for another specialised area within or outside the health service, or you could start a new business from scratch, building on your health knowledge.

Be aware of your personal strengths, career and job preferences, motivation and priorities in life. Think how you want to balance time spent on work and leisure, and work and income. Understand what levels of responsibility, challenge and interaction with other people suit your personal style.

Is a portfolio career right for you? Try doing a SWOT analysis

You could undertake a SWOT analysis of your situation, working out the strengths, weaknesses, opportunities and threats (SWOT) (*see* page 44) as in Box 6.2. Doing the SWOT analysis with someone else can give you a more objective perspective.

Box 6.2: SWOT analysis of you converting to a portfolio career

Possible strengths and opportunities of a portfolio career:

- potentially better paid part-time posts (e.g. expert posts)
- more time can be spent with colleagues (e.g. NHS politics, management, educational posts)
- flexible working enables you to fit in other commitments
- opportunities for creativity (e.g. educational post, writing, projects, leadership)
- combine work and hobby (e.g. travel, sports, writing)
- more public respect for your achievements (e.g. high profile post, project manager)
- instigate change (e.g. NHS politics, government post, project management)
- potentially increased job satisfaction and variety

Possible weaknesses and threats:

- reduced patient contact and less influence on decision making, because of your lower profile in your current practice or organisation, may not suit you
- you may earn less in a non-clinical post
- as locum or sessional worker you may have no income while on holiday, or if you are sick or training
- financial insecurity
- seeking sessional or consultancy work continually can be personally draining
- making lesser contributions to NHS pension if in non-NHS post
- strain on your relationships with your partner or children maybe, if you travel away from home a lot or are focused on work even in your home life

What attributes should you possess to make a success of a portfolio career?

Enthusiasm and interest are key. You need to be flexible and willing to take the risks involved, if you are giving up a secure full-time post. You will have to cope with change and uncertainty unless you settle quickly into regular work. Good time management is essential if you are going to juggle several diverse jobs.

It is easier to make a go of a portfolio career if you have an established expertise that others seek. This might be a clinical expertise backed by a postgraduate qualification and experience, or an educational qualification and background, for instance. You might be an experienced project manager or facilitator who can transfer their skills between settings and challenges.

How to decide what options to explore

Reflect on what you are looking for from your work:

- the kind of work you enjoy – routine, exciting, prestigious
- the setting in which you want to work – community, hospital, rural, urban, travel
- the type of people for whom you want to care – ages and characteristics of patients
- the type of people with whom you want to work – whether in a small team or big organisation
- the extent of patient contact that suits you
- the level of income you consider (a) essential and (b) desirable
- the working hours, holidays, study leave: how the hours fit with your current state and future domestic plans
- opportunities for parallel career interests such as research, writing, education, consultancy, private work or work-related hobbies
- the extent of professional autonomy and responsibility you want
- in fact, your career anchors (*see* Chapter 1).

You should also take account of:

- the details of any training required – hours, practical difficulties, examinations
- the job prospects of alternative career paths: the opportunities for you to progress.

Then find out about the range of opportunities that match with what you want out of your portfolio career. Look out for job adverts in the usual way or local circulars. Seek out more careers information. Sound out people in your networks.

How much of the regular job should you give up? Persuading your trust or practice

Reducing to a part-time commitment may be difficult – others at work probably will not like any suggested change where you seem to be less available. Some full-time staff still scorn the part-time or assistant worker for 'shirking' the responsibility of full-time work. They might advertise for another part-time member of staff or arrange a job-share, appoint a nurse practitioner or make do with less doctor or manager time. Every trust's or practice's circumstances will be different.

If you are a GP partner or other independent contractor with the NHS such as a dentist, optometrist or pharmacist, you should establish a fair way of calculating the financial arrangements such that you keep externally earned pay for work done completely outside your core working hours in your own time, so long as the additional work does not impinge on the practice.

Good planning is key, so that you opt for a mix of jobs that suit you, and end up with a portfolio of posts that together give you a fulfilling career. Anticipate any barriers that may impede your career progress or make the sustaining of your portfolio untenable. Work through the five-point plan in Activity 6.3 and adapt it as your own action plan.

Activity 6.3: Five-point action plan for making your portfolio career happen

1 Take stock – of the advantages and drawbacks
2 Review what opportunities there are
3 Match your abilities and circumstances to the job options
4 Negotiate with your manager or colleagues to reduce your current work commitment
5 Make a well considered change to your portfolio career

7

What now? Making the jump

Kay Mohanna

Watch out for the right job

You should keep a watch for advertisements for jobs you might like to do in the near or distant future, even if you're not ready to move on yet. That way, you are preparing yourself for your future career path. You are making sure that you will have sufficient qualifications and experience by the time you feel ready to reply to a similar advert.

There has been so much change in the NHS that new types of posts are springing up all the time. Send for a few application packs and look at the job descriptions to get a clearer idea about the various kinds of jobs that are available in your specialty or area, and the essential and desirable criteria making up the person specifications. That will help you to group the posts together, and get an idea of what the advertisers are looking for, in relation to the particular level of seniority at which the posts are pegged. If you are employed by a trust and are a non-medic, the way the post is described in terms of job evaluation and the specific dimensions and their levels of the Knowledge and Skills Framework (KSF) should help you to compare the scope of different posts.

When you are preparing and revising your personal development plan (PDP) you need to bear in mind what additional knowledge, skills and experience you will need, to stand a chance of getting one of the jobs you have your eye on. Negotiate with your line manager, or discuss with your appraiser how you will incorporate the necessary learning or experience within your PDP. Find out how you can prioritise your interests against the competing learning needs arising from your current job or expected service developments.

Completing the application form

For most posts, selection will be made by an appointments committee on the basis of an application form (including a curriculum vitae (CV)), references, and interview, with or without a presentation.[1,2] Each post and appointments committee will be different, so there are no hard and fast rules.

Generally at least two people from the appointments committee will shortlist the four or five (sometimes fewer, other times more) candidates for interview. They should have done the shortlisting independently of each other, each comparing your application letter and CV against the person specification linked to the job description. They will read your cover letter too, gauging your enthusiasm, and whether you have shown that you understand what the job is about. What are you trying to sell a future employer about yourself? Describe these strengths in a succinct way. Craft your cover letter to address the nature of the post for which you are applying. Address your letter to a named person, if the name of the senior person connected with the appointment is given.

Your CV

Your CV is your shop window. It has to be good enough to get you shortlisted for that interview so that your undoubted qualities have an opportunity to shine through. Looks are all important, so make sure that your application has a well designed layout that will catch the eye of those doing the shortlisting, especially if you're expecting lots of competition for the post(s) you are going for. Pay attention to the following points.

- A poorly organised CV may be interpreted as evidence of poor communication skills. Think carefully about the layout. Ensure that your strengths are clearly presented. Do not be modest.
- Do not go into too much detail about your earlier years, but make sure that all dates are correct and there are no gaps to account for. If you have had a career break be prepared to justify it.
- Tailor your CV for each application. Identify important information in the advertisement and the person specification, and draw the attention of the people shortlisting to your suitability by summarising your key strengths on a front page. That's what the appointment committee really want to know.
- Consider a competency-based CV. Explain how it is that you are competent for the job you have applied for. This does not concentrate on what posts you have held, but what you have achieved. So it might state for example, that you learnt basic surgical principles during your surgical house job, performed operations X, Y and Z unassisted in a casualty post, have been on a minor surgery course and are now on the approved list for minor surgery. Or a nurse applying for a senior management post might describe the competencies she has gained in people and project management in her pathway through a series of hospital and general practice nursing jobs.
- Resist the temptation to say 'please see CV' if an application form is required to be filled in.
- Spelling mistakes are inexcusable with word processed CVs. Get someone to proof read it for you for other errors. These will be distracting and detract from the content of your application. Consider asking a senior colleague for their comments on whether you have organised your CV in a way that is expected for a particular specialty.
- Keep your CV short and to the point – do not pad it out with unnecessary words or be repetitive. Use action words like 'achieved' to start your sentences where you are describing your experience.

Preparing for the interview

Once shortlisted you must be prepared to capitalise on your achievements. Increasingly, candidates are asked to prepare a presentation on a given topic. This is your opportunity to give a slick demonstration of your communication, organisational and information technology skills.

- Speak to the present incumbent if it is a hospital or primary care post, and the key personnel in the department or practice. Consider meeting the chair or a director of the local trust. Try to find out what the local issues are for the trust and the department or practice.
- Consider visiting the workplace you would be working in if you were successful in your application. Is the waiting room full? Are the receptionists flustered? Look at the standard of maintenance; does a tatty building mean a tatty organisation too?
- Find out who is on the interview panel by ringing the administrative assistant or person whose contact details are given in the letter inviting you for interview, if that letter does not include the information. If you know who is on the panel and their posts, you can anticipate the type of questions they will pose at interview and prepare well.
- Ask for a copy of the annual report of the trust, or practice. It will help you to gauge the size and strength of the organisation, as well as give you ammunition to ask intelligent questions. Is there a development plan with an associated educational plan?
- Decide why you want the post, what you want from the post and what compromises you can make.
- Plan some questions that show your interests. What are the research opportunities like for example, or the continuing professional development facilities? What opportunities are there for diversification to gain and practise other skills?
- Do not assume the interview panel can remember the details in your CV – or have read it even. Emphasise your strengths and experience as you reply to their questions.
- Prepare a short aide-mémoire or handout that you can leave behind, so that they can remember which candidate you were. Nothing too ostentatious though. If you use PowerPoint in your presentation, your handout should include a copy of your slides (in colour) for each panel member, as well as a copy of any other achievement you want them to note.

The big day

By the time you are called for an interview, members of the panel have already seen something in your application that makes them want to take a look at you. Remember this if you think you are starting to flounder, and regain your positive mental attitude. The better prepared that you are the less likely it is that someone can bowl you a 'googly'.

Do not antagonise interview panels by questioning or even arguing a point. But consider how you will fit into an organisation that does not think in a similar way to you. The interview may be the first time that you realise that you and your potential employers or the organisation are incompatible. Be honest with yourself and the interview panel.

Some of the points below should be relevant to your situation; not all will be applicable for all interviews. The interview is designed to test your reactions under stress to a certain extent. Often the interviewer is more interested in the way you handle a question than the content of what you say.

- Dress to impress. Old fashioned advice? You are trying to sell yourself as competent and capable. Having said that, be yourself and express your personality; you must feel comfortable.
- The first few questions will be designed to put you at your ease and settle your nerves. Make eye contact, smile and look interested. If you can remember the names of anybody as they are introduced to you that is a bonus. Avoid saying 'It is all there in my application form'. These are your starters-for-ten.
- Some questions are predictable. Have answers for:
  - why do you want to work here?
  - what are your strengths ...
  - ... and weaknesses? If they ask this try to think of a weakness that you have adjusted for e.g. 'I'm not very good at time management, but I am learning to delegate more'
  - what skills will you bring to the team?
  - what is your vision for the way the post will develop?
- Be up to date with current health issues. Read the journals and newspapers. Have a view.
- Do not be put off by apparently biased questions. It is unlikely that the interviewer is really sexist or ageist or discriminating in other ways. You may have misunderstood. Sometimes humour helps.
- Some questions can be unnerving if you do not know the answer. The best thing is to admit your ignorance but say how you would go about finding out 'That is an interesting question'; 'I would have to look that up/ask someone'.
- Find the balance between thinking before you speak and thinking out loud if you are unsure about an answer. Interviewers may be interested in how you approach a question even if you do not know instantly what they are driving at. If you do put your foot in it, do not dig any deeper. It is okay to say 'Actually now I think about it, that's a daft answer' and have another stab at it. Or ask them to rephrase the question for you (but only do that once in an interview).
- Honesty and integrity show through. Do not try to second guess the 'correct' answer. Politics are unlikely to be overtly discussed, but issues such as rationing of healthcare, private healthcare, how the lottery money should be spent, may be. Say what you think and try to justify it.
- Some interviewers specialise in unusual questions, especially in general practice. Have a think about:
  - what book are you reading at the moment?
  - which famous people, past or present, would you like to invite to dinner?
  - who was more important: Florence Nightingale or Marie Curie?
  - if you were stuck in a lift with the Health Minister, what would you say?

The presentation

Think of a presentation as an opportunity not a threat, as a challenge rather than a problem. Try and see it from the interviewers' perspectives. It is a very boring task to interview half a dozen people who may be very similarly qualified on paper. In a presentation you are in control and you can stress your strengths to the panel. The

Institute of Management has published many books that can help with this type of task.[3]

- Your talk should be concise and well prepared. You should understand the task and stick to it.
- Time yourself and keep to the time limit. It is surprising how long those short notes you wrote can last. (Conversely, you may find you deliver the talk much faster on the day.)
- Try to make the presentation interesting with appropriate use of visual aids. Only use technology that you are familiar with; today is not the day to learn about PowerPoint presentations if you have never done that before. If you are inexperienced or unsure, a few well designed overheads delivered slowly with a strong message will be more effective than an all-singing, all-dancing presentation, even if the latter is more eye-catching. It will also be less easy for you to make a mistake.
- Practise presenting out loud at home. Ask a family member or colleague to hear you practise and give you feedback.
- Give yourself plenty of time to arrive and set up. Ask whoever is organising the interviews if you can give them a copy of your presentation on a disc or CD before the event, so that they preload it for you.

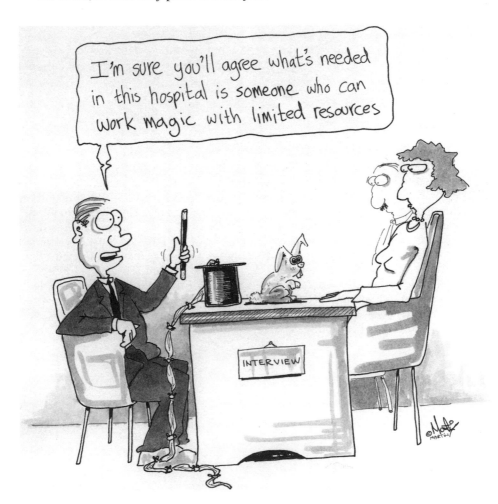

Your golden opportunity

At the end of nearly every interview comes the question 'Is there anything you would like to ask us?'. This should not be met merely with a sigh of relief that the interview is nearly over, but grasped with both hands as your opportunity both to show your enthusiasm for the post and to find out some more details.

- You could ask about standards or developments: e.g. do they do regular audit, how are problem issues dealt with, or what plans they have for development?
- How is the workload shared and what are the outside commitments of those in the department or practice? For instance, are consultants on lots of committees leaving the incoming doctor to do a disproportionate share of routine work; do others in the team work flexibly?
- Is there a team approach or is there a sense of autocratic leadership? This can be a tricky area to uncover the truth. A question such as 'who makes the final decision if there is disagreement?' may be revealing.
- What is the potential to maximise income either by private practice or outside jobs in general practice (if you are an independent contractor)?
- What is the availability of study leave? How are study leave and holidays organised? Is backfill generally available for staff on booked leave? Are there restrictions on how many can be away at once?
- What is the information technology infrastructure and support like?
- Does the department or practice have links with others for support or educational activities?

Referees

People usually think hard about whom they will nominate as referees. It makes sense to choose someone whom you think will speak or write well of you. However the influence a referee can have is often exaggerated.

The main reason for providing references is to ensure that there is objective confirmation of a candidate's history. A reference generally says more about the referee than the applicant. References should be used to confirm what has been discovered through the shortlisting and interviewing processes. So usually a panel will not look at the references until after the interviews have been conducted; some organisations only obtain references for the preferred candidate after the interviews have been held. While the qualitative information within a reference may be able to make a difference if two candidates are very close, they are the least important part of the application process. A poor reference is not much help to the candidate, but a good reference is not much help to the panel.

References

1 Cook M (1998) Traditional ways of selecting medical staff. *BMJ Classified.* **316, 7 March:** 2–3.

2 Cook M (1998) New approaches to selecting medical staff. *BMJ Classified.* **316, 14 March:** 2–3.

3 Jay R (1995) *Effective Presentation. The Institute of Management Foundation.* Pitman Publishing, London.

8

Making a logical plan to develop your career

Ruth Chambers

This book is packed with good advice about planning your career. In the past, you may have leafed through journals and newspapers looking at job adverts or dreamt of developing your skills to further your career. But you may not have made any positive plans for doing so until now. You may not have had the confidence to believe that you too could succeed. You may have felt ground down by work and too tired to make plans let alone study for new qualifications. After returning from holiday you might vow to take on all sorts of career development activities in future – but when back at work you soon become tired and apathetic about progressing your career again.

Does this sound familiar? You need to reflect on why your good resolutions to improve your career have failed in the past. It is probably because carrying out your resolutions was a lot more complex a matter than simply making the resolutions. Other factors may have intruded that you had not foreseen. Your willpower might not have been sufficient, you may not have had the skills or time or money for your new promised way of life, or you may have mistakenly presumed that others at home or work would support you in making your planned career changes.

Why not regard your career development as a project, and use the logical framework (log frame) approach to help you to succeed in carrying out your good resolutions? This type of project management approach sets out what activities, achievements and purpose you need to achieve your goal(s). The log frame handles the complex nature of making and undertaking an action plan to improve your career and set specific goal(s). It helps you to analyse your weaknesses and guides you to consider the assumptions that you are making – in the details of your plan of action or in pursuing your goals. This approach helps you to realise the interactions between what you can do for yourself, and external factors that either enhance, or hinder your plans.

With the log frame you will set out realistic milestones and decide in advance how you will monitor your progress. It helps you to:

- organise your thinking about your career
- relate your planned activities to the results you can expect
- set performance indicators for yourself
- allocate responsibilities for yourself and to others – at work and at home.

Advantages of a logical framework

The logical framework has been used for project planning for decades.[1] Development agencies have adopted the approach for planning and monitoring overseas programmes. Recently it has been used by the health service for planning and evaluating health action zone projects.[2,3]

The approach will force you to consider the assumptions you are making in setting out your action plan. You will be able to monitor your progress and pre-empt obstructions to your plans. The log frame is an aid to thinking rather than a series of procedures to which you slavishly adhere. The framework will help you to concentrate on the operational aspects of your career 'project' – and complete the who, when, why and how components.[1]

The structure of the log frame consists of a 4 × 4 matrix. The rows represent the project objectives and the means to achieve them (vertical logic). The columns indicate how you can verify that you have achieved your objectives (horizontal logic) and the assumptions that you are making. A simple outline is given in Table 8.1.

Table 8.1:   Simple 4 × 4 matrix of a logical framework

	Summary	Indicators	Verification	Assumptions and risks
Goal				
Purpose				
Outcomes (intermediate achievements)				
Activities				

A simplified overview of an example of a completed logical framework is given in Table 8.2. You can see how someone who undertakes activities 1.1, 1.2, 1.3 and 1.4 achieves outcome 1 in the section above: their 'completed career development plan'. Someone who undertakes activities 2.1, 2.2 and 2.3 should achieve outcome 2, an 'additional clinical qualification'. Someone undertaking activities 3.1, 3.2, 3.3, 3.4 and 3.5 should achieve outcome 3: 'become competent in a particular special clinical interest area'. Once attained, these three outcomes should lead to the purpose, 'maintain competence in post with special clinical interest', and in turn to the ultimate goal, to 'achieve a fulfilling career'.

The assumptions and risks described in the far right-hand column of Table 8.2 are all pertinent to the activities, outcomes, purpose and goal of the rows alongside them. As you go on, more activities are built in to anticipate these assumptions and risks, so as to minimise the barriers to progressing from the planned activities to the outcomes and upwards to the purpose and goal. The middle column captures some examples of ways in which you can monitor your interim and overall achievements, while completing the preliminary activities and overall logical framework plan.

Table 8.2: Simplified example of a completed log frame to achieve a fulfilling career (with middle two columns merged to simplify the overview of completed log frame)

	Summary	Indicators/ Verification	Assumptions and risks
Goal	Achieve a fulfilling career	Remain at work in NHS	You are fulfilled by your new area of clinical expertise
Purpose	Maintain competence in post with special clinical interest	Agreed reports of competence	You receive sufficient support to continue ongoing training
Outcomes	1 Completed career development plan	1 Completed career plan, PDP approved	1.1 You and others have skills to complete career plan 1.2 Career plan is relevant to you, and your aspirations
	2 Additional clinical qualification obtained	2 Award/ clinical qual.	2.1 Qualification is relevant to clinical interest area
	3 Become competent in a particular special clinical interest area	3 Feedback from service users/trust	3.1 Training course and clinical supervision are sufficient 3.2 You can show competence
Activities	1.1 Obtain careers guidance	1 Attend careers guidance Action plan from audit of job satisfaction Map competencies/ trust strategy	1.1 Careers guidance available is well informed and impartial
	1.2 Review own commitments and career aspirations, audit own job satisfaction		1.2 Able to review commitments – other input from colleague, able to audit job satisfaction
	1.3 Make career plan		1.3 Able to write a career plan
	1.4 Agree competency of new post		1.4 Risks: no agreement between trust/ professions re competency
	2.1 Compose PDP, justifying special clinical interest, discuss at appraisal	2 PDP has action plan re clinical interest/ service plans Log of work	2.1 Able to compose a balanced PDP and justify clinical priority, supported by appraiser
	2.2 Incorporate expert clinical role into service delivery		2.2 Trust/practice will extend services and recognise you as expert

Continued

2.3 Practise new skills		2.3 Clinical placement exists
3.1 Apply for support for course fee, find resources for cover and study	3 Obtain cover & bursary for career plan	3.1 Can obtain support for fee, capacity to cover
3.2 Locate appropriate training for clinical award	Suitability of course verified	3.2 Quality and scope of training course can be determined
3.3 Attend training course	Evidence of performance after training and clinical placements	3.3 Spare capacity on course
3.4 Work in supervised clinical placements in course		3.4 Clinical placements exist, are well structured and relevant
3.5 Trust or university extends numbers of clinical placements with support		3.5 Insufficient capacity or type of clinical placements

Now have a go yourself at making your own logical framework

If you like this approach and want to work through a detailed version, building it up stage by stage, please follow the logic in Table 8.3 and progress through Tables 8.4, 8.5, 8.6 and 8.7 to Table 8.8. Then take time out to map out your own verifiable action plan in a similar way.

If you want to look at other related but different examples of log planning such as beating stress at work in a health setting, see how a goal stated as 'To minimise stress in my working life' works out in Chambers R, Schwartz A and Boath E (2003) *Beating Stress in the NHS: how to do it.* Radcliffe Medical Press, Oxford or look at how 'To achieve successful revalidation' works out in Chambers R, Wakley G, Field S and Ellis S (2003) *Appraisal for the Apprehensive.* Radcliffe Medical Press, Oxford.

The vertical logic

- *Step 1*: define your overall goal – the reason for you undertaking the 'career project'. This is your ultimate objective. Phrase this in your own words. An example might be 'to achieve a fulfilling career'.
- *Step 2*: define the purpose of your 'career project'. This is what you expect to have achieved within your timescale. An example might be 'to maintain competence in a post with a special clinical interest'. It keeps your career project more streamlined if you only have one purpose. Although you will try your best, it will not be entirely within your control to achieve the purpose of your project. In the example given in this chapter, you might be unable to influence the primary care trust to invest in

that clinical interest area by employing you or providing the resources for making the special clinical services available to patients, even though you and others have undertaken the preliminary work that demonstrates the need.

- *Step 3*: define the outcomes for achieving the purpose of your 'career project'. These are what you want the project to achieve – the specific end results that will be achieved when the planned activities are carried out. We've called them 'intermediate achievements' in Table 8.1 as they are on the way to gaining your purpose, and thereafter your overall goal. An example might be to 'become competent in the special clinical interest area'. Achieving the outcomes should be within your control.
- *Step 4*: define the activities that you will undertake in order to achieve each outcome, and what resources are available. Activities define how you will carry out your project. Examples might be 'to obtain careers guidance or make a career development plan'. You should expect to undertake three to seven activities for every outcome you hope to accomplish (*see* Table 8.4 for an example).

The log frame structure is based upon the concept of cause and effect. The vertical logic is based on a sequence of causal relationships starting from the bottom upwards. There is a logical relationship between activities and outcomes, outcomes and the purpose, the purpose and the goal. So **if** specific activities are carried out **then** certain outcomes will be produced. If the outcomes you describe are produced, then the declared purpose will be achieved. If the purpose is achieved, your goal should be attained.

So from the bottom upwards:

GOAL

then ↑

if PURPOSE

then ↑

if OUTCOMES

then ↑

if ACTIVITIES

The horizontal logic

Horizontal logic underlies the way you measure the effectiveness of your career plan. Specify how you will measure progress for each of the four levels of the vertical logic: the activities, outcomes, purpose and goal. Use concrete terms rather than vague measures, as far as possible, as tangible indicators of progress. These indicators should have the following qualities:

- clearly describe how the achievement of the activity, outcome or purpose contributes to the success of your overall careers project
- focus on what is important for the purpose or overall goal
- clearly relate to the activity, outcome, purpose or goal with which they are associated

- be of sufficient number and in enough detail to measure activities, outcomes, purpose and goal adequately
- be specific to an activity, outcome, purpose or goal
- be able to be verified: two independent observers should measure achievement in the same way.

The indicator might be direct (e.g. the actual clinical interest post you attain) or indirect (e.g. your job satisfaction when practising the clinical interest post). These indicators should be SMART:

- **S**pecific
- **M**easurable
- **A**chievable
- **R**ealistic
- **T**ime limited.

Then decide how you will verify that all the specified indicators have been achieved. You might gather simple data as part of your careers project, or refer to sources of information such as reports, official documents, notes of meetings or an appraisal review.

Important assumptions and risks

Once you have mapped out the vertical logic starting with the activities and following those through outcomes and purpose to the overall goal, test out the cause and effect relationship. **If** these activities are carried out, **then** you will achieve these outcomes. **If** you register for a postgraduate clinical award, **then** you will be competent in the special clinical interest area ... you can see that the case is crumbling – there are missing links. You cannot assume that the postgraduate award will automatically lead to a special clinical interest post. You will have to do more than simply register for the postgraduate award; you will have to learn new skills and complete any assignments satisfactorily and then practise the new skill in varying circumstances to become competent and improve with feedback from others about your technique. You have been assuming that registering for and attending a training course is all that you need to do, whereas in actual fact besides activities such as practising the skills learnt, you should have undertaken linked activities such as prioritising learning about those clinical skills, located an appropriate training course, created time to go, justified the course fees etc.

You know that it is very unlikely that your plans will go forward without a hitch, but that doesn't stop you assuming that you will progress smoothly. In reality, things crop up to obstruct or delay your progress that you have not expected or anticipated.

The assumptions that you describe in your log frame include factors or conditions that could affect your progress with your career development project over which you have no, or limited, control. For the overseas development projects with which the log frame has been used, these might include external factors such as unexpected bad weather or an earthquake.

For you, trying to achieve a fulfilling career, examples of major external factors beyond your control are the government changing priorities away from the special clinical interest area, or the illness of a colleague necessitating you taking on their basic work at the expense of working time spent on your special clinical interest area. More minor assumptions might be the extent of co-operation that is forthcoming from others in your family or your colleagues at work if you are proposing to reduce your income or spend time away from your workplace gaining further qualifications. These will affect whether you are able to undertake many of the career development activities you plan, or achieve the planned outcomes or purpose in your log frame.

As well as the unexpected factors that might spoil your plans, you may be assuming too much. It may be that you have insufficient knowledge and skills for the career development activities you envisage. Or, you might not have forecast the extent of qualifications, time or income needed to implement your plans, for instance.

There may be other risks to your planned timetable too. You may not have thought through the consequences of your plans – such as how you will manage to do your everyday work as well as that of the new special clinical area, in line with your plans. Or you may not have predicted the new stress-provoking factors that might arise from your revised weekly schedule when trying to fit in additional clinical work or studying for further qualifications.

Getting started

Read through the series of steps below and work through the thinking behind how we have put the log frame together. Before you start, note down all the people who will have some influence on the progress or viability of your career development plan. They might include:

- colleagues at work
- managers in your department or practice or trust
- staff at work to whom you delegate work
- people who delegate work to you
- people for whom you are responsible
- your spouse/partner or family at home
- relatives who are dependent on you etc.

You will need to anticipate how they will influence your career plan – to enhance or limit your progress. So, consider how they will interact with you and include them in the activities of your log frame, or in the assumptions that you make. You will be taking account of their influence, by harnessing their help or preventing them from obstructing you, in the nature of the activities that you include in your plan.

The worked example that we develop below illustrates the processes that you need to adopt to make up a log frame. The contents of the example log frame are an illustration of the thinking behind a log frame and are not prescriptive. You should use the evolving framework as a guide rather than lift the example 'off the peg' for your own requirements. Much of the learning and benefits from a log frame arise from the preparatory work in putting it together and thinking through the factors that are individual to you that will enhance or prevent your progress. They will be peculiar to you, your trust or practice, networks of people and your circumstances.

We have not included every detail about possible assumptions or potential risks that might occur during such a careers project plan or even the numerous activities that you could undertake. To do so would have resulted in such an extent of back--ground detail that it would be difficult for you as the reader to distinguish 'must do' information from 'could do' detail. You will be able to include more information about risks and assumptions yourself – the columns of a completed log frame that is undertaken over a year or more often stretches to over three or four sides of A4 paper.[4]

Table 8.3:   Step 1 of building up the log frame to achieve a fulfilling career: your first attempt at planning your vertical logical pathway

	Summary	*Indicators*	*Verification*	*Assumptions and risks*
Goal	Achieve a fulfilling career			
Purpose	Maintain competence in post with special clinical interest			
Outcomes (intermediate achievements)	Completed career development plan			
	Additional clinical qualification			
	Become competent in a particular special clinical interest area			
Activities	Obtain careers guidance			
	Make a career development plan			
	Register for a postgraduate clinical award			
	Apply for funding/bursary for postgraduate course fee			

Look again at these activities and outcomes: **If** you apply for funding or a bursary for your course fee and register for a postgraduate award **then** ... what? The outcomes described in Table 8.3 were about obtaining the additional clinical qualification and planning for and being competent in that clinical area. There are *no* intermediary steps in the list of activities for converting the information gathered in the career review or protecting time for study, or creating opportunities to practise your novice skills in a clinical setting, and *no* specific outcomes for each activity – so you need to add some more activities – as we do in **bold** in Table 8.4.

Numbering the outcomes and the activities linked to them will help you to see how **if** you undertake certain activities **then** you will achieve specific outcomes – as in Table 8.4.

Now that you are starting to get the vertical logic in place, you should start thinking out what assumptions you have been making, and whether there are any potential risks associated with your logical plan. Once you have recognised these you may have to add other activities in, to minimise the effects of previously unforeseen external factors. This is the stage when you should be anticipating problems that could interrupt the progress of your project action plan. You may have a blind spot about these possible problem areas, so you could usefully discuss the preliminary thinking of your project plan with someone else such as your partner or a friend, who might point out weaknesses you have not yet recognised, or give you information about possible external influences of which you were unaware.

Table 8.4: Step 2 of building up the log frame to achieve a fulfilling career: linking activities with outputs

	Summary	Indicators	Verification	Assumptions and risks
Goal	Achieve a fulfilling career			
Purpose	Maintain competence in post with special clinical interest			
Outcomes	1 Completed career development plan 2 Additional clinical qualification 3 Become competent in a particular special clinical interest area			
Activities	1.1 Obtain careers guidance **1.2 Review own work commitments and career aspirations** **1.3 Carry out audit of own job satisfaction** 1.4 Make a career development plan			
	2.1 Compose personal development plan (PDP) **2.2 Justify and prioritise special clinical interest in PDP taking into account personal, trust/ NHS perspectives** **2.3 Discuss PDP at appraisal or performance review with appraiser, clinical supervisor or manager and trust; agree plan to prioritise special clinical expertise** **2.4 Continue to liaise with trust/ practice about how, when and where to incorporate expert clinical role into service delivery** **2.5 Practise newly gained skills in clinical setting, under supervision** **2.6 Get feedback from supervisor and patients about performance in expert clinical role**			
	3.1 Locate appropriate training course **3.2 Work with trust/colleagues to find resources to provide cover for study time** 3.3 Apply successfully for funding or bursary for course fee			

Continued

3.4 Register for relevant
postgraduate clinical award
3.5 Attend training course
3.6 Work in supervised clinical
placements as part of course

Look at the additions in **bold** in Table 8.5 to see some examples of assumptions that
you might be making. You can see that as you think through how you are going to
undertake those activities and turn them into outcomes, some gaps are appearing –
you may be assuming you already possess the knowledge and skills to compose a PDP,
or that you are capable of undertaking a review of your job satisfaction. You may

Table 8.5: Step 3 of building up the log frame to achieve a fulfilling career: adding in
assumptions about your planned activities

	Summary	Indicators	Verification	Assumptions and risks
Goal	Achieve a fulfilling career			
Purpose	Maintain competence in post with special clinical interest			
Outcomes	1 Completed career development plan 2 Additional clinical qualification 3 Become competent in a particular special clinical interest area			
Activities	1.1 Obtain careers guidance			**1.1 Careers guidance available is well informed and impartial**
	1.2 Review own work commitments and career aspirations			**1.2 Able to review commitments – other input available such as from partner or colleague**
	1.3 Carry out audit of own job satisfaction			**1.3 Able to undertake audit of job satisfaction**
	1.4 Make a career development plan			**1.4 Able to write a career plan**
	2.1 Compose personal development plan (PDP)			**2.1 Able to compose a balanced PDP around learning cycle**
	2.2 Justify and prioritise special clinical interest in PDP taking into account personal, trust/NHS perspectives			**2.2 Able to justify why special clinical area is priority: e.g. lack of current expertise, service need**

2.3 Discuss PDP at appraisal or performance review with appraiser or clinical supervisor or manager and trust; agree plan to prioritise special clinical expertise	**2.3 Appraiser/ manager are supportive of career plan and prioritisation of special clinical area**
2.4 Continue to liaise with trust/ practice about how, when and where to incorporate expert clinical role into service delivery	**2.4 Trust/practice prepared to extend clinical services; recognise/welcome you as potential clinical expert**
2.5 Practise newly gained skills in clinical setting, under supervision	**2.5 Suitable clinical mentor and placement exists/is accessible**
2.6 Get feedback from supervisor and patients about performance in expert clinical role	**2.6 Supervisor and patients give constructive/ positive feedback that is useful and relevant**
3.1 Locate appropriate training course	**3.1 Quality and scope of training course can be determined**
3.2 Work with trust/colleagues to find resources to provide cover for study time	**3.2 There is spare workforce capacity to provide cover; amount of study time required is reasonable**
3.3 Apply successfully for funding or bursary for course fee	**3.3 Application is successful or you can pay fee yourself**
3.4 Register for relevant postgraduate clinical award	**3.4 Spare capacity exists on selected clinical award/course**
3.5 Attend training course	**3.5 You/colleagues remain healthy so you attend course, and do not cover sick colleagues**
3.6 Work in supervised clinical placements as part of course	**3.6 Clinical placements exist locally, have capacity, are well structured, provide relevant experience and teaching**

assume that you will find an appropriate course locally, but there is nil available when you seek it. Or you might mistakenly assume that your trust or practice will support you in your endeavours to develop a new clinical area with resources to cover your absence on study leave or delivering the clinical skill outside your usual role. You will then add more activities in the summary column to address these assumptions, as we do later in Table 8.6.

Table 8.6: Step 4 of building up the log frame to achieve a fulfilling career: add more activities to anticipate the 'risks' arising from previously planned activities and assumptions

	Summary	Indicators	Verification	Assumptions and risks
Goal	Achieve a fulfilling career			
Purpose	Maintain competence in post with special clinical interest			
Outcomes	1 Completed career development plan 2 Additional clinical qualification 3 Become competent in a particular special clinical interest area			
Activities	1.1 Obtain careers guidance			1.1 Careers guidance available is well informed and impartial
	1.2 Review own work commitments and career aspirations			1.2 Able to review commitments – other input available such as from partner or colleague
	1.3 Carry out audit of own job satisfaction			1.3 Able to undertake audit of job satisfaction
	1.4 Make a career development plan			1.4 Able to write a career plan
	1.5 Attend workshop to learn about career planning **1.6 NHS sets up careers guidance services that include non-medical/NHS careers guidance experts**			**Risks** **1.5 Entirely NHS directed career guidance/planning limits scope**
	2.1 Compose personal development plan (PDP)			2.1 Able to compose a balanced PDP around learning cycle
	2.2 Justify and prioritise special clinical interest in PDP taking into account personal, trust/NHS perspectives			2.2 Able to justify why special clinical area is priority: e.g. lack of current expertise, service need
	2.3 Discuss PDP at appraisal or performance review with appraiser or clinical supervisor or manager and trust; agree plan to prioritise special clinical expertise			2.3 Appraiser/ manager are supportive of career plan and prioritisation of special clinical area
	2.4 Continue to liaise with trust/ practice about how, when and where to incorporate expert clinical role into service delivery			2.4 Trust/practice prepared to extend clinical services; recognise/welcome you as potential clinical expert
	2.5 Practise newly gained skills in clinical setting, under supervision			2.5 Suitable clinical mentor and placement exists/is accessible
	2.6 Get feedback from supervisor and patients about performance in expert clinical role			2.6 Supervisor and patients give constructive/positive feedback that is useful and relevant

	Risks
2.7 Trust organises training for managers and workforce about potential of practitioners with special clinical interests	**2.7 Delivery of the clinical expertise is inappropriate in primary care setting; defence societies do not provide indemnity cover**
2.8 Trust or professional organisations formally approach medical defence societies to check out potential cover for practitioners with special clinical interests	
3.1 Locate appropriate training course	3.1 Quality and scope of training course can be determined
3.2 Work with trust/colleagues to find resources to provide cover for study time	3.2 There is spare workforce capacity to provide cover; amount of study time required is reasonable
3.3 Apply successfully for funding or bursary for course fee	3.3 Application is successful or you can pay fee yourself
3.4 Register for relevant postgraduate clinical award	3.4 Spare capacity exists on selected clinical award/course
3.5 Attend training course	3.5 You/colleagues remain healthy so you attend course, and do not cover sick colleagues
3.6 Work in supervised clinical placements as part of course	3.6 Clinical placements exist locally, are well structured, provide relevant experience and teaching
	Risks
3.7 Trust and/or local university extends numbers of clinical placements with support network and training for clinical mentors	**3.7 Insufficient capacity or type of clinical placements**

The type of risks that may arise are that: you will waste your time attending a clinical skills course that does not fit your, or the trust's or practice's needs; you cannot find the right course pitched at an appropriate level for you that is held at a convenient time and is affordable. Other areas of risk will include: staff numbers remaining stable so that you can be released for study leave or the new expert clinical work; that no significant new government directives etc are issued that overturn your and others' priorities; no crisis occurs at your workplace such as some calamity like a flood or fire.

So, the next step is to add yet more activities to anticipate the risks that you realise could happen, to reduce the likelihood of them occurring and obstructing your progress with your plan. The risks and activities given in **bold** in Table 8.6 are illustrative of a variety of risks that might occur, and activities that you might adopt to minimise the effects of these risks on your progress to achieving a happier and more balanced life.

The next step is to move on to specify the assumptions that you are making about attaining your outcomes, your purpose and overall goal. We have started this process in the additions given in **bold** in Table 8.7, but in reality you would have far more to add in these sections. You need to think of any external factors that are needed, or might prevent you attaining the outcomes or the long-term sustainability of your goal or purpose, for your careers project to be successful.

Table 8.7: Step 5 of building up the log frame to achieve a fulfilling career: adding various assumptions you are making about expected outcomes, your purpose and goal, and adding more activities to diminish the likelihood of potential risks occurring

	Summary	Indicators	Verification	Assumptions and risks
Goal	Achieve a fulfilling career			**You are fulfilled by your new area of clinical expertise**
Purpose	Maintain competence in post with special clinical interest			**You receive sufficient support to continue ongoing training**
Outcomes	1 Completed career development plan			**1.1 You and others have the knowledge and skills to complete a career plan** **1.2 The career plan is relevant to you, and your aspirations for clinical expertise and work situation, practice or trust**
	2 Additional clinical qualification			**2.1 The clinical qualification is relevant to the particular clinical interest area and is more than a theory award**
	3 Become competent in a particular special clinical interest area			**3.1 The training course and clinical supervision are sufficient for you to become competent** **3.2 There is a way for you to demonstrate competence**
Activities	1.1 Obtain careers guidance			1.1 Careers guidance available is well informed and impartial
	1.2 Review own work commitments and career aspirations			1.2 Able to review commitments – other input available such as from partner or colleague

1.3 Carry out audit of own job satisfaction
1.4 Make a career development plan

1.5 Attend workshop to learn about career planning
1.6 NHS sets up careers guidance services that include non-medical/ NHS careers guidance experts
1.7 Describe and agree with trust expected competency of new post in particular clinical area
1.8 Trust creates new posts in particular clinical area and agrees service delivery across primary/secondary care settings
2.1 Compose personal development plan (PDP)

2.2 Justify and prioritise special clinical interest in PDP taking into account personal, trust/NHS perspectives

2.3 Discuss PDP at appraisal or performance review with appraiser or clinical supervisor or manager and trust; agree plan to prioritise special clinical expertise
2.4 Continue to liaise with trust/ practice about how, when and where to incorporate expert clinical role into service delivery

2.5 Practise newly gained skills in clinical setting, under supervision

2.6 Get feedback from supervisor and patients about performance in expert clinical role

2.7 Trust organises training for managers and workforce about potential of practitioners with special clinical interests
2.8 Trust or professional organisations formally approach medical defence societies to check out potential cover for practitioners with special clinical interests
2.9 Workforce Development Directorates (WDDs), deaneries etc train educationalists and managers in careers information and guidance skills

1.3 Able to undertake audit of job satisfaction
1.4 Able to write a career plan

Risks
1.5 Entirely NHS directed career guidance/planning limits scope

2.1 Able to compose a balanced PDP around learning cycle
2.2 Able to justify why special clinical area is priority: e.g. lack of current expertise, service need
2.3 Appraiser/ manager are supportive of career plan and prioritisation of special clinical area
2.4 Trust/practice prepared to extend clinical services; recognise/welcome you as potential clinical expert
2.5 Suitable clinical mentor and placement exists/is accessible
2.6 Supervisor and patients give constructive/positive feedback that is useful and relevant

Risks
2.7 Delivery of the clinical expertise is inappropriate in primary care setting; defence societies do not provide indemnity cover

Continued

2.10 NHS organises career planning workshops for all NHS staff

3.1 Locate appropriate training course	3.1 Quality and scope of training course can be determined
3.2 Work with trust/colleagues to find resources to provide cover for study time	3.2 There is spare workforce capacity to provide cover; amount of study time required is reasonable
3.3 Apply successfully for funding or bursary for course fee	3.3 Application is successful or you can pay fee yourself
3.4 Register for relevant postgraduate clinical award	3.4 Spare capacity exists on selected clinical award/course
3.5 Attend training course	3.5 You/colleagues remain healthy so you attend course, and do not cover sick colleagues
3.6 Work in supervised clinical placements as part of course	3.6 Clinical placements exist locally, are well structured, provide relevant experience and teaching
	Risks
3.7 Trust and/or local university extends numbers of clinical placements with support network and training for clinical mentors	3.7 Insufficient capacity or type of clinical placements
3.8 Trusts work with universities to commission courses and awards, accrediting competencies of those delivering clinical services	
3.9 WDDs and deaneries run ongoing training and support for practitioners with special clinical interests	

You will need to think about the 'potential risks' that are likely to arise too. The assumptions that you are making and the risks you anticipate should trigger you to add extra activities and outcomes to your right-hand column in real life. We have *not* added any more extra activities or outcomes here to anticipate assumptions and risks of the outcomes, purpose and goal in our example log frame in Table 8.7 for the sake of simplicity, but you will certainly have to do so to take adequate measures to ensure your smooth progress with your careers plan.

You may, for instance, assume that you can protect time for study in a regular way, whereas in reality there will be unforeseen circumstances that interrupt your plans. There will be a potential risk, for instance, that in protecting time for a special new interest for you, new time pressures are created for the rest of the work team.

Your final step will be to describe the indicators for all your activities, outcomes, purpose and goal – and what will be the means by which you can verify that you have achieved them. You should add a timescale too for each indicator. The indicators should be do-able and worthwhile.

The examples of indicators added to Table 8.8 are given in **bold**. They show how someone might do their best to fix appropriate indicators and give examples of how the indicators might be verified.

Table 8.8: Step 6 of building up the log frame to achieve a fulfilling career: adding indicators and the means of verification of progress for your planned activities, outcomes, purpose and goal as examples here

	Summary	Indicators (examples)	Verification (examples)	Assumptions and risks
Goal	Achieve a fulfilling career	**You have job satisfaction from your balanced career most of the time**	**1.1 Successive appraisals/ performance reviews reports reflect job satisfaction** **1.2 You remain working in NHS until normal retirement age**	as for Table 8.7
Purpose	Maintain competence in post with special clinical interest	**1.1 Positive feedback from service users**	**1.1 No or few patient or colleague complaints about service you provide; unsolicited and requested positive feedback reports**	as for Table 8.7
		1.2 You and others in team/trust feel confident about your expertise in special clinical interest area	**1.2 Successive demonstrations of competence – in own learning portfolio**	
		1.3 Agreed balance of time/ responsibilities at work, on expert clinical area/general post	**1.3 Renewal of contracts in special clinical interest area by trust**	
Outcomes	1 Completed career development plan	**1.1 Career development plan drawn up by self or recommended career plan template completed**	**1.1 Completed career development plan discussed with careers guide who confirms realism, balance in appended report**	as for Table 8.7
		1.2 and 1.3 PDP completed and submitted to CPD or lead tutor	**1.2 PDP and career development plan overlap in demonstrable ways** **1.3 CPD or lead tutor officially approves PDP each year as justifying resources requested or pledged**	
	2 Additional clinical qualification	**2.1 Complete course or award** **2.2 Pass test for clinical qualification**	**2.1 and 2.2 Certificate of attainment of clinical qualification**	

Continued

	3 Become competent in a particular special clinical interest area	**3.1 Positive feedback from service users**	**3.1 Positive feedback report about the extent of your clinical expertise given by clinical supervisor for annual appraisal**	
		3.2 You and others in team/trust feel confident about your expertise in special clinical interest area	**3.2 Log of application of clinical skill and record of no or few critical incidents or adverse events**	
Activities	1.1 Obtain careers guidance	**1.1 Attend recommended number of careers guidance sessions in time period**	**1.1 Diary of careers guidance sessions and reflections about discussions**	as for Table 8.7
	1.2 Review own work commitments and career aspirations	**1.2 Time spent reviewing current work situation and career options**	**1.2 Notes of strengths and weaknesses, threats and opportunities of own career and various career options**	
	1.3 Carry out audit of own job satisfaction	**1.3 Audit of job satisfaction within 2 months**	**1.3 Audit record with reflections appended**	
	1.4 Attend workshop to learn about career planning	**1.4 Attended workshop on career planning within 2 months**	**1.4 Certificate of attendance at workshop & template of career plan**	
	1.5 Make a career development plan	**1.5 Drawn up career development plan after careers guidance**	**1.5 Record of career development plan included in own portfolio**	
	1.6 NHS sets up careers guidance services that include non-medical/ NHS careers guidance experts	**1.6 Trust/deanery strategy agreed by 6 months to establish careers support with generic careers experts**	**1.6 Brochure of careers advice and guidance services and contact details for range of experts**	
	1.7 Describe and agree with trust expected competency of new post in particular clinical area	**1.7 Mapping out of competencies of practitioners with special clinical interests**	**1.7 Competencies of various new clinical posts published e.g. on trusts' websites**	
	1.8 Trust creates new posts in particular clinical area and agrees service delivery across primary/secondary care settings	**1.8 Trust workforce strategy linked to service delivery plans by end of planning year**	**1.8 Trust's approved workforce and service delivery plans available to public**	
	2.1 Compose personal development plan (PDP)	**2.1 PDP drawn up**	**2.1 PDP approved at annual appraisal (each year) at work**	
	2.2 Justify and prioritise special clinical interest in PDP taking into account personal, trust/ NHS perspectives	**2.2 Action plan for learning about clinical interest coincides with priority in one of trust's strategic plans**	**2.2 Action plan in PDP and trust's strategic plans with links indicated**	

2.3 Discuss PDP at appraisal or performance review with appraiser or clinical supervisor or manager and trust; agree plan to prioritise special clinical expertise

2.3 PDP central to appraisal/ performance review

2.3 Appraiser's/ manager's report supports prioritisation of learning/training in relation to special clinical area

2.4 Continue to liaise with trust/practice about how, when and where to incorporate expert clinical role into service delivery

2.4 Feed views to practice/trust about extension of services relating to special clinical interest area

2.4 Notes of papers submitted and documentary reports of meetings etc

2.5 Practise newly gained skills in clinical setting, under supervision

2.5 Take up clinical opportunities created with supervisor

2.5 Log of clinical practice in special clinical interest

2.6 Get feedback from supervisor and patients about performance in expert clinical role

2.6 Invite feedback from patients, supervisor and colleagues about performance

2.6 Feedback slips about performance with reflective review of strengths and weaknesses revealed by feedback

2.7 Trust organises training for managers and workforce about potential of practitioners with special clinical interests

2.7 Invite national expert to address managers and local workforce about potential and practical issues of creating practitioners with special clinical interests

2.7 Flyer for the event and evaluation slips including requests for further training

2.8 Trust or professional organisations formally approach medical defence societies to check out potential cover for practitioners with special clinical interests

2.8 Trust writes to defence societies before advertising new posts for practitioners with special clinical interests

2.8 Trust's and defence society's correspondence or notes of meetings if relevant

2.9 WDDs, deaneries etc train educationalists and managers in careers guidance skills

2.9 WDDs and deaneries run training for providers of careers advice and guidance across region in current financial year

2.9 Flyers for training events, application forms, attendance lists etc

2.10 NHS organises career planning workshops for all NHS staff

2.10 WDDs and deaneries and trusts run career planning workshops and invite all staff

2.10 Flyers for training events, application forms, attendance lists etc reflect equitable access from staff groups

3.1 Locate appropriate training course

3.1 Liaise with local universities to identify range of courses; search online for courses farther afield

3.1 Curriculum and handbook for course you and trust/ practice deem most appropriate

Continued

3.2 Work with trust/colleagues to find resources to provide cover for study time	**3.2 Apply to trust and practice colleagues for funds and cover for specific study days in 12-month period**	**3.2 Confirmation letter from trust or practice manager to provide cover for study days in protected time with reasonable terms and conditions**
3.3 Apply successfully for funding or bursary for course fee	**3.3 Apply for funding or bursary within one month of completing career plan**	**3.3 Letter from trust or other sponsor confirms funding or bursary for at least part of course fees**
3.4 Register for relevant postgraduate clinical award	**3.4 Application for postgraduate award submitted soon after course identified**	**3.4 University or other body confirms your place on course, that you meet admission criteria**
3.5 Attend training course	**3.5 Attend training course study days**	**3.5 Attend at least 90% of study days of training course**
3.6 Work in supervised clinical placements as part of course	**3.6 Attend and work in clinical placements required by course**	**3.6 Attend and work in clinical placements required by course for at least 90% of expected time**
3.7 Trust and/or local university extends numbers of clinical placements with support network and training for clinical mentors	**3.7 Trust and/or local university reviews capacity of current clinical placements and recruits and trains new clinical mentors**	**3.7 Trust and/or university recruits at least 90% of mentors needed and trains and supports 100% of those**
3.8 Trusts work with universities to commission courses and awards, accrediting competencies of those delivering clinical services	**3.8 Staff responsible for education/training in trusts meet with WDD to discuss needs to commission new accredited courses**	**3.8 Notes of meetings and plans, documents to inform learning strategies, and agreed strategies for workforce development**
3.9 WDDs and deaneries run ongoing training and support for practitioners with special clinical interests	**3.9 WDDs and deaneries set up support groups themed for practitioners with special clinical interests with training calendars**	**3.9 Good attendance (90% of those invited) at ongoing training activities of various support groups**

Concluding your logical plan for your career development

Now that you have finished mapping out your log frame, you should refine it and discuss it with a colleague or tutor or mentor to see if it is realistic or if there is something else that you have not thought of. Seek out experts in the field in which you hope to develop your expertise. Discuss the assumptions and risks you have thought of with people in your practice or trust that can help you to overcome any problems or likely barriers to your plans.

Find out if there are people with the expertise and time to give you careers information, guidance or counselling – depending on what level of help and enablement you require. If you are a nurse, for example, maybe your clinical supervisor, mentor or practice educator would be appropriate (*see* Chapter 4).

Decide how often you are going to review your log frame. A six-monthly review, say, should enable you to keep a track of your progress. The extent to which you and others meet the indicators should give you a good idea about how you are getting on. You may then realise too that there are additional assumptions and risks that you have not previously thought of or addressed. Add yet more activities in to address them!

References

1 Coleman G (1987) Logical framework approach to the monitoring and evaluation of agricultural and rural development projects. *Project Appraisal*. **2**: 251–9.

2 Centre for Rural Development and Training (2000) *A Guide for Developing a Logical Framework*. University of Wolverhampton, Wolverhampton.

3 Jacobs B (2001) *Logical Framework and Performance Management*. North Staffordshire Health Action Zone, Stoke-on-Trent.

4 Spender A and Chambers R (2001) *Logical Framework Plan for Teenwise Project*. Staffordshire University, Stoke-on-Trent (unpublished).

And finally: Seven steps to getting on – your checklist

Wendy Garcarz

All these tools and approaches may be confusing you – you may be thinking you can have too much of a good thing. Here's a checklist of seven steps for you to really crystallise the actions you can take.

Step 1: know yourself

- Review and update your CV; it is a snapshot of your career.
- Reflect on what makes you tick, your leadership and decision-making styles, the extent to which you are a team player.
- Be clear about what is important to you in your career.

Step 2: understand what you want

- How much of a challenge do you want?
- How much do you want to follow other people's guidance or lead?
- How much money do you want or need?
- What kind of work/life balance suits you?

Step 3: know where you are

- Have a good understanding of your achievements and skills.
- Know your strengths and weaknesses.
- Understand what your career anchors are.

Step 4: be clear where you want to go

- Check out the options and opportunities open to you.
- Compare what is on offer with your responses to steps 1 and 2 above.

Step 5: mind the gap

- Analyse the gap between where you are now and the variety of options for where you want to be.

Step 6: plan how to get there

- Have a range of strategies to bridge that gap in your career plan.
- Develop a realistic action plan with contingencies for if or when your ideal career path does not work out.

Step 7: get supporters

- Find a mentor.
- Develop a network outside your immediate colleagues of others who are or could be important to you or informative about your future career.

Appendix 1 :
Generic careers support information for all in the NHS

National organisations

*   *Chartered Institute of Personnel and Development*, 151 The Broadway, London SW19 1JQ. Tel: +44 (0)20 8612 6200. www.cipd.co.uk
    Services provided include promotion of programmes, management consultation and training, guides on career management in organisations and counselling at work. Provides references for reports, articles and books about careers support.
*   *International Health Exchange/Red R*, 1 Great George Street, London, SW1P 3AA. Tel: +44 (0)20 7233 1100. www.ihe.org.uk
    This is a charity assisting aid and development organisations to recruit qualified health professionals, through recruitment, training and works with agencies and individuals worldwide.
*   *Learndirect*, PO Box 900, Manchester, M60 3LE. Tel: +44 (0)800 100 900. www.learndirect-advice.co.uk
    A national advice organisation offering general careers advice and information. You can call an advice line to discuss career options.
*   *NHS Alliance*, Goodbody's Mill, Albert Road, Retford, Notts DN22 6JD. Tel: +44 (0)1777 869080. www.nhsalliance.org
    Representative organisation of primary care.
*   *NHS Careers*, PO Box 376, Bristol BS99 3EY. Tel: +44 (0)845 60 60 655. www.nhscareers.nhs.uk
    Website gives information and national/local contact details.
*   *National Primary and Care Trust Development Programme (NatPaCT)*, 2nd floor, Blenheim House, West One, Duncombe Street, Leeds LS1 4PL. Tel: +44 (0)113 254 3800 www.natpact.nhs.uk
    Provides organisational development support to primary care trusts.
*   *NHS Professionals*. Recruitment line: +44 (0)845 6060 345. www.nhsprofessionals. nhs.uk
    Aims to maximise the potential of doctors, nurses and corporate staff with support and flexibility to meet their own personal needs. Has guidance on flexible career schemes, training for lifelong learning etc.
*   *Salomons Centre for Leadership and Management Development*, Broomhill Road, Southborough, Tunbridge Wells, Kent TN3 0TG. Tel: +44 (0)1892 507633. www.salomonsclmd.co.uk
    Able to provide psychometric and other instruments for self-awareness (Myers Briggs, MBTI, ABLE etc). Also specialise in the education, training and development of health professionals.
*   *Society for Academic Primary Care (SAPC)*, 4 Manor Farm Barns, Church Lane, Charlton-on-Otmoor, Oxon OX5 2UA. Tel: +44 (0)1865 331839. www.sapc.ac.uk
    Aims to promote excellence in research and education in general practice and primary healthcare.

Publications/websites

- Schein E (1993) *Career Anchors. Discovering your real values.* Pfeiffer and Co, California. www.pfeiffer.com
- Schein E (1996) *Career Anchors.* Trainer's Manual. Pfeiffer and Co, California. www.pfeiffer.com
  Two workbooks on helping to identify career choices.
- Department of Health *Improving Working Lives Standards.* Department of Health, London. www.dh.gov.uk/assetRoot/04/07/40/65/04074065.pdf
- *Health Service Journal.* www.hsj.co.uk
  Weekly publication provides general information, courses and conferences and appointments section.
- *NMAP.* http://nmap.ac.uk
  Provides internet resources for nursing, midwifery and allied health professionals.

Appendix 2:
Careers information for doctors

Expert/specific careers support

- *BMJ Careers Focus*, BMA House, Tavistock Square, London WC1H 9JR. Tel: +44 (0)20 7383 6125. www.bmjcareers.com
  Provides careers information and advice for medics through personal articles. Advertises jobs, courses; advice for overseas applicants and disabled doctors. Has chronic illness matching scheme.
- *Medical Forum*, 24 Woodlands, Overton, Hants RG25 3HN. Tel: +44 (0)705 007 7171. www.medicalforum.com
  Provides careers guidance, professional growth and personal development for medical and dental professions. Offers personalised careers guidance and resources to learn how to compose career plan.
- *Medical Practitioners' Union*, 40 Bermondsey Street, London SE1 3UP. Tel: +44 (0)20 7939 7000. www.mpunion.org.uk
  A medical organisation that recognises the political issues of poverty, environments, living and working conditions, which need to be addressed if the health of the population is to be improved.
- *Medical Women's Federation*, Tavistock House North, Tavistock Square, London WC1H 9HX. Tel: +44 (0)20 7387 7765. www.medicalwomensfederation.co.uk
  Aims to advance the personal and professional development of women in medicine. Updates and informs members of changes affecting the medical profession and women's health issues. Offers members advice and support in their careers.
- *NHS Professionals*. Recruitment line: +44 (0)845 6060 345. www.nhsprofessionals.nhs.uk
  Aims to maximise the potential of all available doctors, with the support and flexibility to meet their own personal needs. Gives guidance on flexible career schemes, training for lifelong learning etc.

National organisations

- *Association for the Study of Medical Education (ASME)*, 12 Queen Street, Edinburgh EH12 1JE. Tel: +44 (0)131 225 9111. www.asme.org.uk
  ASME is a membership organisation for doctors and educators from any clinical specialty and level. Offers careers guidance and personal development for healthcare professionals.
- *British International Doctors' Association*, 316A Buxton Road, Great Moor, Stockport SK2 7DD. Tel: +44 (0)161 456 7828.
- *British Medical Association*, BMA House, Tavistock Square, London WC1H 9JP. Tel: +44 (0)20 7387 4499. www.bma.org.uk
  The BMA represents doctors from all branches of medicine all over the UK, keeping members up to date with clinical and other medical issues. The science and

education department provides information on the different agencies and advisers you may wish to contact in seeking solutions to career problems.

- *General Medical Council (GMC)*, Regent's Place, 350 Euston Road, London NW1 3JN. Tel: +44 (0)845 357 8001. www.gmc-uk.org
  The GMC's aim is to maintain the standards of doctors that the public expect.
- *Medical Research Council*, 20 Park Crescent, London W1B 1AL. Tel: +44 (0)20 7636 5422. www.mrc.ac.uk
  The MRC's major forms of support are research grants and awards for training and research career development, covering all stages of a research career.
- *National Association of Sessional GPs (NASGP)*, PO Box 188, Chichester, West Sussex PO19 2ZA. Tel: +44 (0)1243 536428. www.nasgp.org.uk
  Offers general support to GP non-principals around their careers.
- *Royal College of Anaesthetists*, 48–49 Russell Square, London WC1B 4JY. Tel +44 (0)20 7813 1900. www.rcoa.ac.uk
- *Royal College of General Practitioners (RCGP)*, 14 Princes Gate, London SW7 1PU. Tel: +44 (0)20 7581 3232. www.rcgp.org.uk
  RCGP faculties might provide careers support.
- *Royal College of Obstetricians and Gynaecologists*, 27 Sussex Place, Regents Park, London NW1 4RG. Tel +44 (0)20 7772 6200. www.rcog.org.uk
- *Royal College of Paediatrics and Child Health*, 50 Hallam Street, London W1W 6DE. Tel +44 (0)20 7307 5600. www.rcpch.ac.uk
- *Royal College of Physicians*, 11 St Andrew's Place, Regents Park, London NW1 4LE. Tel +44 (0)20 7935 1174. www.rcplondon.ac.uk
- *Royal College of Physicians and Surgeons of Glasgow*, 232–242 St Vincent Street, Glasgow G2 5RJ. Tel +44 (0)141 221 6072. www.rcpsglasg.ac.uk
- *Royal College of Psychiatrists*, 17 Belgrave Square, London SW1X 8PG. Tel +44 (0)20 7235 2351. www.rcpsych.ac.uk
- *Royal College of Surgeons of Edinburgh*, Nicolson Street, Edinburgh EH8 9DW. Tel +44 (0)131 527 1600. www.rcsed.ac.uk
- *Royal College of Surgeons of England*, 35–43 Lincoln's Inn Fields, London WC2A 3PE. Tel +44 (0)20 7405 3474. www.rcseng.ac.uk
- *Royal Institute of Public Health*, 28 Portland Place, London W1B 1DE. Tel +44 (0)20 7580 2731. www.riph.org.uk

Publications/websites

- *British Medical Journal (BMJ)*, BMJ Careers Focus section, BMJ, BMA House, Tavistock Square, London WC1H 9JR. Tel: +44 (0)20 7387 4499. www.bmj careers.com, http://bmj.bmjjournals.com/careerfocus
- *Doctors.net.uk* www.doctors.net.uk
  Qualified doctors or medical students can access the site. Offers information and jobs.
- *Employing Doctors and Dentists*, Chamberlain Dunn Associates, Gothic House, 3 The Green, Richmond TW9 1PL. Tel: +44 (0)20 8334 4500. www.chamberlaindunn.com
  Newsletter published 10 times a year, for those involved in recruiting, employing and managing medical and dental staff. Has informative articles on progress in dentistry plus news on conferences and publications.
- Baker M and Chambers R (eds) (2000) *A Guide to General Practice Careers*. RCGP, London.

- British Medical Association (1998) *Medical Careers: a general guide.* BMA, London.
- British Medical Association (2003) *Signposting Medical Careers for Doctors.* BMA, London.
- Chambers R, Mohanna K and Field S (2000) *Opportunities and Options in Medical Careers.* Radcliffe Medical Press, Oxford.
- MacDonald R (ed) (2003) *My Beautiful Career.* BMJ Careers workbook. BMJ, London.
- Ward C and Eccles S (2001) *So You Want to be a Brain Surgeon?* (2e). Oxford University Press, Oxford.
- Whitehouse AB (2003) *Careers Information Pack.* West Midlands Deanery, Birmingham.

Appendix 3:
Careers information for nurses

Expert/specific careers support

- *Nursing and Midwifery Council*, 23 Portland Place, London, W1B 1PZ. Tel: +44 (0)20 7637 7181. www.nmc-uk.org
- *Royal College of Nursing Immigration Advice Service*. Tel: +44 (0)845 456 6766. Confidential appointment-based service for overseas nurses and nursing students. Offers advice on a wide range of immigration and work permit issues.
- *Royal College of Nursing Learning Zone*. www.rcn.org.uk
  Has a careers section – job profiles, advice on developing career planning skills, where to apply for courses and funds, and search for jobs.
- *Royal College of Nursing Nurseline*, Tel: +44 (0)20 7647 3463. nurseline@rcn.org.uk, www.rcn.org.uk
  Independent advice and information service for nurses and midwives plus provides support and help on personal matters or hardship.

National organisations

- *British Nursing Association*, The Colonnades, Beaconsfield Close, Hatfield, Hertfordshire AL10 8YD. Tel: +44 (0)800 581691 (freephone). www.bna.co.uk
  Has a job shop and career section for registered nurses and care assistants – updated weekly.
- *Community Practitioners' and Health Visitors' Association*, 40 Bermondsey Street, London SE1 3UD. Tel: +44 (0)20 7939 7000. www.msfcphva.org
  Offers careers advice on an *ad hoc* basis to its members. Gives advice on career changes for those in primary and community care. Information on health visitor training. Offers information packs for district nurses, school nurses and practice nurses on interview techniques plus up-to-date reading material to prepare them for interview. Offers courses on leadership.
- *Royal College of Nursing*, 20 Cavendish Square, London W1G 0RN. Nurseline: +44 (0)20 7647 3463. www.rcn.org.uk
  Offers telephone information and guidance e.g. change of direction within nursing. Information on educational opportunities. Help with job applications, CV and interview skills. Will search databases on courses for professional development.
- *UNISON Health Care Service Group*, 1 Mabledon Place, London WC1H 9AJ. Tel: +44 (0)845 355 0845. www.unison.org.uk
  Offers information on careers, qualifications and training.

Publications/websites

- Department of Health (2001) *Making a Difference in Primary Care: the challenge for nurses, midwives and health visitors*. Department of Health, London. www.dh.gov.uk

- Kenkre J and Foxcroft DR (2001) *Career Pathways for Research Nurses.* Research and Development Co-ordination Centre, Manchester University, Manchester. www.man.ac.uk/rcn/rs/career.htm
- *Nurse Scribe.* www.enursescribe.com
  Lifelong learning resources for nursing students, staff nurses, nurse educators and nurse authors. Comprehensive site – American bias but has British resources as well. Has a careers development archive.
- *Nurses' Network.* www.nursesnetwork.co.uk
  This is a new interactive online resource made for nurses by nurses. Offers help, information, advice, chat and research.
- *Nursing Standard.* www.nursing-standard.co.uk
  Good website offering information on professional development, courses, events, links, jobs and careers advice and information.
- Sanderson J (1993) *Career Development for Nurses – opportunities and options.* Scutari Press, Middlesex.
- *Nursing Times.* www.nursingtimes.net
  Weekly publication, plus website. Has sections on careers, jobs, plus archive articles on primary care and management.

Appendix 4: Careers information for allied health professionals (dietitians, physiotherapists, speech and language therapists, occupational therapists, podiatrists)

National organisations

- *British Dietetic Association*, 5th Floor, Charles House, 148/9 Great Charles Street, Queensway, Birmingham B3 3HT. Tel: +44 (0)121 200 8080. www.bda.uk.com
  No careers pack but has information on continuing professional development, clinical placement and details about working as a dietitian.
- *Chartered Society of Physiotherapy*, 14 Bedford Row, London WC1R 4ED. Tel: +44 (0)20 7306 6666. www.csp.org.uk
  Good search feature to find references to careers in physiotherapy. Has two publications online: *Physiotherapy* monthly journal, *Frontline* fortnightly magazine.
- *College of Occupational Therapists* and *British Association of Occupational Therapists*, 106–114 Borough High Street, Southwark, London SE1 1LB. Tel: +44 (0)20 7357 6480. www.cot.co.uk, www.baot.co.uk
  No specific careers section. The *British Journal of Occupational Therapists* is online.
- *Health Professions Council (HPC)*, Park House, 184 Kennington Park Road, London SE11 4BU. Tel: +44 (0)20 7582 0866. www.hpc-uk.org
  This is the independent, UK-wide regulatory body responsible for setting and maintaining standards of professional training, performance and conduct.
- *Royal College of Speech and Language Therapists*, 2 White Hart Yard, London SE1 1NX. Tel: +44 (0)20 7378 1200. www.rcslt.org
  Has information on return to practice, postgraduate education etc. The college has two periodicals/newsletters online – the *Bulletin* and *Supplement*.
- *Society of Chiropodists and Podiatrists*, 1 Fellmonger's Path, Tower Bridge Road, London SE1 3LY. Tel: +44 (0) 20 7234 8620. www.feetforlife.org
  Good website with lots of information on careers in podiatry.

Publications/websites

- *AHP Bulletin*. AHP Branch, Wellington House, 135–155 Waterloo Road, London SE1 8UG. www.doh.gov.uk/ahpbulletin/index.htm
  Staff can receive the *AHP Bulletin* directly by email each month by emailing their details to DH-Test-Emails@doh.gsi.gov.uk.
- Department of Health (2000) *Allied Health Professionals – building careers.* Department of Health, London. Tel: +44 (0)8701 555 455. www.dh.gov.uk
  Provides information for all allied health professionals.

- Department of Health (2002) *Improving Working Lives for the Allied Health Professions and Healthcare Scientists.* Department of Health, London. www. doh.gov.uk

Appendix 5:
Careers information for optometrists

National organisations

- *Association of Optometrists*, 61 Southwark Street, London SE1 0HL. Tel: +44 (0)20 7261 9661. www.assoc-optometrists.org
  Provides services and representation to promote and protect its members.
- *Federation of Ophthalmic and Dispensing Opticians*, 113 Eastbourne Mews, London W2 6LQ. Tel: +44 (0)20 7258 0240. www.fodo.com
  Represents the business interests of registered opticians.
- *General Optical Council*, 41 Harley Street, London W1G 8DJ. Tel: +44 (0)20 7580 3898. www.optical.org
  Regulatory body for optometrists.
- *The College of Optometrists*, 42 Craven Street, London WC2N 5NG. Tel: +44 (0)20 7839 6800. www.college-optometrists.org
  Professional, scientific and examining body for optometry in the UK. Also includes research and career information.

Publications/websites

- *Optometry Journal.* www.optometryonline.net
  Weekly journal. Vacancies page.

Appendix 6:
Careers information for pharmacists

National organisations

- *Amicus Health*, MSF Centre, 33–37 Moreland Street, London EC1V 8HA. Tel: +44 (0)20 7505 3000. www.amicustheunion.org
  Has a section for employee pharmacists in the community. Vacancies page.
- *Association of the British Pharmaceutical Industry*, 12 Whitehall, London SW1A 2DY. Tel: +44 (0)20 7930 3477. www.abpi.org.uk
  Has a section on education, training and careers.
- *College of Pharmacy Practice*, 28 Warwick Row, Coventry CV1 1EY. Tel: +44 (0)24 7622 1359. www.collpharm.org.uk
  Provides post-registration training and continuing professional development.
- *Guild of Healthcare Pharmacists*. www.ghp.org.uk
  The Guild contributes to pharmaceutical education at postgraduate level.
- *National Pharmaceutical Association*, Mallinson House, 38–42 St. Peter's Street, St Albans, Herts AL1 3NP. Tel: +44 (0)1727 832161. www.npa.co.uk
  Has a section on careers for pharmacists, pharmacy technicians, dispensary assistants and medicine counter assistants.
- *Royal Pharmaceutical Society of Great Britain*, 1 Lambeth High Street, London SE1 7JN. Tel: +44 (0)20 7735 9141. www.rpsgb.org.uk
  No specific vacancies page but offers general information and careers advice.

Publications/websites

- Department of Health (2004) *Improving Working Lives for the Pharmacy Team*. Department of Health, London. www.dh.gov.uk/PolicyAndGuidance/Human ResourcesAndTraining/ModelEmployer/ImprovingWorkingLives/fs/en
- *Pharmaceutical Journal*. www.pharmj.com
  Lots of articles on careers, and educational pages.

Appendix 7:
Careers information for dentists

Expert/specific careers support

- *Medical Forum*, 24 Woodlands, Overton, Hampshire RG25 3HN. Tel: +44 (0)705 007 7171. www.medicalforum.com
  Careers guidance, professional growth, personal development and empowering career management for dentists.

National organisations

- *British Dental Association (BDA)*, 64 Wimpole Street, London W1G 8YS. Tel: +44 (0)20 7935 0875. www.bda-dentistry.org.uk
  Offers general information and careers advice section.
- *Dental Practice Board (DPB) for England and Wales*, Compton Place Road, Eastbourne, East Sussex BN20 8AD. Tel: +44 (0) 1323 433550. www.dpb.nhs.uk
  Works in conjunction with strategic health authorities in England and Wales and aims to maintain practice standards as well as providing refresher courses and training days.
- *Faculty of Dental Surgery at The Royal College of Surgeons of England*, 35–43 Lincoln's Inn Fields, London WC2A 3PE. Tel: +44 (0)20 7405 3474. www.rcseng.ac.uk
  Has information on career grades including advice and guidance for trainers. Covers dental specialties of orthodontics, paediatric and restorative dentistry. Has a vacancies page.
- *General Dental Council (GDC)*, 37 Wimpole Street, London W1G 8DQ. Tel: +44 (0)20 7887 3800. www.gdc-uk.org
  Regulatory body of the dental profession. Has no careers section but offers general information.
- *King's College London*, University of London, Malet Street, London WC1E 7HU. Tel: +44 (0)20 7862 8360/8361/8362. www.londonexternal.ac.uk
  Offers distance learning in specialist areas of dentistry.
- *National Centre for Continuing Professional Education for Dentists (NCCPED)*, 4th Floor, 123 Gray's Inn Road, London WC1X 8TX. Tel: +44 (0)20 7905 1222.
  Supports and evaluates dental educational courses and activities and provides a 'getting back to practice' scheme for those who have taken a career break.
- *Royal Society of Medicine: Odontology Section*, 1 Wimpole Street, London W1G 0AE. Tel: +44 (0)20 7290 3934/3859. www.roysocmed.ac.uk/academ/secodont.htm

Publications/websites

- *British Dental Journal (BDJ)*. www.nature.com/bdj
  The official journal of the British Dental Association. Does not carry a specific section on careers but there are occasional careers articles.
- *Dental Channel*. www.dental-channel.co.uk
  Offers peer-reviewed continuing professional development courses on CD-ROM free of charge.
- *Dental Web*. www.thedentalweb.com
  General information, education features and jobs.
- *Dentistry Magazine*, Dentistry Editorial Department, FMC Ltd, 1 Hertford House, Farm Close, Shenley, Herts. Tel: +44 (0)1923 851750. www.dentistry.co.uk
  Published fortnightly. Has a regular section entitled 'My life, my career', personal profiles.
- *Employing Doctors and Dentists*, Chamberlain Dunn Associates, Gothic House, 3 The Green, Richmond TW9 1PL. Tel: +44 (0)20 8334 4500. www. chamberlaindunn.com
  Newsletter published 10 times a year, for those involved in recruiting, employing and managing medical and dental staff. Has informative articles on progress in dentistry plus news on conferences and publications.
- Kendall B (2001) *Opportunities in Dental Care Careers*. NTC Publishing Group, London.

Appendix 8: Careers information for managers in primary care

Expert /specific careers support

- *Institute of Healthcare Management*, 46 Grosvenor Gardens, London SW1W 0EB. Tel: +44 (0)20 7881 9235. www.ihm.org.uk
  Professional body for managers working in healthcare and health services. Has discussion forums and chat rooms, contacts, news and helpline. Also includes a section specifically for primary care managers and careers information.

National organisations

- *Healthcare People Management Association*, 13a City Business Centre, Lower Road, Rotherhithe, London SE16 2XB. Tel: +44 (0)20 7252 3707. www.hpma.org.uk
  Provides careers information and training.
- *Executive Choice*, Dearden Consulting Ltd, The Gallery Office, Chewton Mendip, near Bath BA3 4NT. Tel: +44 (0)1761 240130. www.dearden.co.uk
  Offers seminars or one-off coaching sessions to prepare for job change. Also offers analysis of Myers Briggs. Also provides counselling service for careers support.
- *Institute of Health Record and Information Management*. www.ihrim.co.uk
  Provides careers information and training.
- *NHS Graduate Schemes*. Tel: +44 (0)870 169 9731. www.futureleaders.nhs.uk
  Provides careers information and training. Information about finance management, general management and human resources.

Publications/websites

- Department of Health (2004) *Working lives – flexing retirement*. Department of Health, London. Tel: +44 (0)8701 555 455. www.dh.gov.uk
  Provides guidance for NHS managers.
- *Primary Care Management*, George Warman Publications (UK) Ltd, Unit 2, Riverview Business Park, Walnut Tree Close, Guildford GU1 4UX.
  Journal for managers in primary care. Published 10 times a year.

Index